How to Survive Hearing Loss

CHARLOTTE HIMBER

Gallaudet University Press
Washington, D.C.

This book is not intended as a substitute for the medical advice of a physician. The reader should regularly consult a physician in matters relating to his or her health, particularly regarding any symptoms that may require diagnosis or medical attention.

Gallaudet University Press, Washington, DC 20002

Published 1989

Printed in the United States of America

Library of Congress Cataloging-in-Publication Data

Himber, Charlotte. 1907–
  How to survive hearing loss / Charlotte Himber.
     p.   cm.
  Includes bibliographical references.
  ISBN 0-930323-60-2 : $17.95
  1. Himber, Charlotte, 1907–   . 2. Aged, Deaf—United States—
Biography. 3. Adjustment (Psychology) I. Title.
HV2534.H56A3   1989
362.4′ 2—dc20   89-38838
                                                                              CIP

Gallaudet University is an equal opportunity employer/educational institution. Programs and services offered by Gallaudet University receive substantial financial support from the U.S. Department of Education.

CONTENTS

FOREWORD

If Charlotte Himber accomplishes only one thing within these pages—if she can eliminate the "denial stage" for Americans with hearing loss—she will be giving a joyous gift to them and their loved ones. Most people who are trapped in the denial stage of hearing loss experience a personal crisis, followed by a time of honest revelation and acceptance; it is a time to admit that by denying their hearing loss they have been lying to others and themselves. Only then will they be able to discuss their hearing loss with friends and loved ones, for the burden of denial and secrecy will have lifted and they will at last be free to accept positive change.

My personal crisis happened in a cow pasture in Petaluma, California, at sunrise on a winter morning, during the filming of a scene for a television movie. The production crews had worked all night to ready this particular farmyard and pasture for a very intricate and expensive scene. Trucks and tractors, hens and geese, actors and extras were set to move on the director's call for "Action!" In the far background, a barn was wired to explode into flames, so this was a one-take-only situation. Everyone was very tense as the final camera checks were completed. My particular moves were simple enough: on the signal, "Action!" I was to start the cows moving, walk through the herd, react to the explosion, and run to my farmhouse. "What a way to make a living," I chuckled to myself as I trudged out into the far pasture to join the twenty or so curious cows.

I looked up and saw the director raise his bullhorn. I waved to indicate that I was in place. All was motionless, silent, ready. But wait! Suddenly the chickens began scattering and the extras started running. "Must be a false start," I thought. "Or did I not hear the magic order, 'Action?'" A painful knot of anxiety twisted in my stomach. "Oh, no," I thought. "Had I missed something important—again?"

As the farmyard came to life and the cameras rolled, something quite unexpected happened. The cows started to move forward without my prodding. Those sad-eyed Guernseys stepped right out, and so did I. Not only did the herd save the production company thousands of dollars, they spared me the embarrassment of having to own up to my hearing impairment.

My little drama within a drama seems quite humorous to me today. In fact, I'm actually grateful it happened because it certainly shocked me out of my denial stage and left me open to the possibility of change. I'm also thankful I was wise enough to recognize and accept fate's message. I realize now that everyone goes through the anxiety and denial I had been living with. I'll be forever indebted to that herd of cows; they moved me to act, and act I did.

I went to the House Institute in Los Angeles for a hearing test. Dr. Ralph Nelson explained to me that I did indeed have a hearing loss, a moderate loss, and he offered several suggestions. I took him up on the hearing-aid evaluation, scouted out a hearing-aid dealer in my neighborhood, and within no time I was sporting as comfortable and attractive a set of Qualitone aids as one could imagine.

My story is not unlike those being told by a rapidly increasing number of people who want to improve the quality of their lives. With hearing aids, we can again feel like full, participating members of society. We hear music more fully now, and we can distinguish the real lyrics—no more guessing at and making up words. Soon after I got my hearing aids, I had a marvelous experience that illustrates my point well.

I have always enjoyed the early music of Bob Dylan and considered myself a Dylan aficionado. But one day, after I recited some Dylan lyrics to our son, my wife corrected me. "No," I insisted, "I probably know this song as well as Dylan himself." To prove it, I dusted off the particular recording and gave it a spin, and then found out I was wrong, and wrong again. Alas, the great Dylan expert of the sixties had feet of clay and ears of tin! But what a treat it was to play the music of my past and hear it fully for the first time. I could only think of how long I had missed the pleasure of the real lyrics because of my fear of what others would think if they knew I had impaired hearing.

How to Survive Hearing Loss helps to allay the fear felt by most people who have lost some hearing ability—that others will dislike or dismiss them because of their hearing loss. Being in a profession in which the understanding of the spoken word is everything, I have been acutely sensitive to this fear and the anxiety it produces. Indeed, it was extremely gratifying to me during a recent episode of "L.A. Law" to have my character, Leland McKenzie, take his hearing aids, which he had tried to hide for fear of being considered old, and turn them into an advantage to win a case. It pleased me to think that millions of hearing and hard-of-hearing people viewed this show. But, millions more need help, too.

More than 20 million Americans have some degree of hearing impairment. Other statistics abound, and one can only guess why, until quite recently, the medical and insurance industries have turned deaf ears to our national suffering and financial waste. They are deaf no longer, thanks in part to positive research efforts and new technological advances that are made known to us practically every day. Congress has also responded by establishing the National Institute on Deafness and Communicative Disorders.

Charlotte Himber persuasively shows us that those with hearing loss can go on with their lives. Her desire that hearing loss no longer remain the "invisible handicap" is becoming a reality. The general public's consciousness about hearing impairments is growing and, in fact, hearing-impaired people are becoming visible in our culture. Former President Reagan set an example for the nation when he frankly admitted his hearing loss and his need to wear hearing aids. Former Surgeon General C. Everett Koop, who is a hearing-aid wearer, has also contributed to the current surge in awareness.

How to Survive Hearing Loss is a landmark achievement. Charlotte Himber has given a warm and honest gift to the American public, and how fortunate we are that she writes with such a fine measure of fact and human understanding. Her clear, lucid explanation of the ear and how it works is unique in the literature, and it adds significantly to this valuable book. This work is all the more vital when we realize that it is her own experience. Like millions of other Americans, Ms. Himber lost her hearing late in life, but unlike them, she has written down her experiences so that others may benefit.

Charlotte Himber deserves much praise for her work. Her superior research and her ability to translate complicated material to the lay person's understanding is a gift beyond measure.

Richard Dysart

PREFACE

When I was a child, my mother used to call me *Träumerin* ("dreamer" in German, her native tongue). "Why can't you listen when I talk to you?" she would ask as I wandered around in our big kitchen, lost in reverie. Fifty years later, an audiologist who tested my hearing reported that I had a sensorineural loss common to the elderly complicated by an additional hearing problem that I must have had as a child.

As I wrote this book, I recalled the Träumerin years along with other, much later occasions when I was criticized for "not listening." Listening, as many episodes in the book demonstrate, is an enervating task for hearing-impaired individuals, an activity that people who lose their hearing can never take for granted.

If my story appears to be merely one person's chronicle, some statistics should convince my readers that many people have firsthand experience with at least some of its features. More than 20 million Americans suffer from some degree of hearing loss. Nearly 20 percent of the population has tinnitus, a ringing in the ears which, if constant, becomes a miserable distraction. Approximately 40 percent of all hearing-impaired people are over sixty-five, and half of them have an impairment in both ears. Their number is so large that everyone is affected directly or indirectly. Surely, the tribulations of so many, and the consequences for all of society, should be documented. From the early years, when the handicap is still invisible, to the time when it becomes a serious impairment with dire results, education is needed to ensure that the widespread repercussions of a hearing loss will be better understood.

By study, research, and interviews with audiologists, otologists, and speech pathologists, I gained a broad knowledge of the subject. My personal experiences illustrate the process of hearing deterioration in people as they mature. As I learned to accept my loss, I formed the resolve to help others escape from the bondage of secrecy and to enlist their cooperation in surmounting the universal prejudice against our invisible handicap. Having been an editor and writer for most of my working life, I found it natural to approach the task by writing a book.

The past three years have been rich and exciting for me, a period of growth as I learned about the remarkable engineering of the human ear. But the most fulfilling time came in the final months when I followed the intensification of research and computer technology, and the rise of national advocacy on behalf of hearing-impaired people, developments which presage a bright future for the millions of us who are hard of hearing.

Thanks to My Mentors, Advisors, and Friends: For professional guidance, interviews, assistance in conducting workshops on coping with hearing loss, criticism of the manuscript, and responses to numerous telephone calls as I checked and rechecked the technical sections, I thank: Michele Carpenter, clinical audiologist at the Hear Center in Port St. Lucie, Florida; Benjamin Dawsey and Jenny Edgemon, audiologists in Spartanburg, South Carolina; Kathleen McKenzie, coordinator, Spartanburg County Hearing Handicapped Program; Gayle Chaney, director of audiology,

South Carolina School for the Deaf and Blind; the staff of the New York League for the Hard of Hearing—Jane Madell, director of audiology, Ruth R. Green, administrator, Joshua Gendel, director of technical services, and Barbara deLeeuw, director of mental health services; Michie O'Day, chapter coordinator at the National Self Help for Hard of Hearing People, in Bethesda, Maryland; the Shepherd's Center, a senior citizens' community center in Spartanburg, whose staff of dedicated volunteers cooperated with me in promoting and planning the workshops; Daniel Malamud, a clinical psychologist and colleague at New York University, who coached and counseled me when we jointly taught courses in self-understanding and interpersonal relationships and thereby helped me acquire the skills and insights I needed to lead community workshops; the reference librarians of the Spartanburg County Library, who devoted hours to completing searches for me and who enlisted the cooperation of librarians throughout South Carolina; the National Council of YMCAs, where I received professional training in developing and conducting seminars for both staff and constituency, leading participants in personal growth, risk taking, and the dynamics of group interaction; Harry Himber, my brother-in-law, an attorney and editorial purist, who reviewed and supervised the typing of the final draft; and Pamela Scanlon Liska, who delayed her vacation to finish typing the manuscript on schedule; Elaine Costello, director, and Ivey B. Pittle, managing editor, of the Gallaudet University Press, whose patience and encouragement provided a lifeline that sustained me during the anxious months of preparation; and especially my husband, Louis Himber, who read and reviewed every page of each of the five drafts for three years, assumed more than his share of domestic duties, and settled for dinners of noodles and cheese so that I could be free to work, and Susan Baker, my daughter, an excellent editorial reviewer, who introduced me to several of her professional colleagues in Spartanburg, counseled me, and helped me research and write about the technical aspects of audiology. Susan helped me to exercise tact and restraint in my writing and supported me with patience and love.

How to Survive Hearing Loss

INTRODUCTION

A Daughter's Tale

Are you wearing your hearing aid, Mom?''

"Not just now."

"Well, for heaven's sake, Mom, will you *please* put it on?"

"I will, I will," she promised with a deep sigh and a smile of resignation.

I had been drawing up my marketing list while she was visiting in our home, and I had just asked her—twice—if she needed anything. She's eighty-nine. She has a severe hearing loss and many other physical problems common at her age. Now she closed her eyes and catnapped. I waited, pencil poised, until she opened them again.

"Did you ask me something?" she requested mischievously, revived now and innocently attentive.

"Your hearing aid," I pleaded, with a poke at my own ear. "Where is it?"

"In my purse. I put it there after the concert last night. I like it quiet after all that listening."

"Why aren't you wearing it now? You *know* you miss a lot when you don't."

"That's true. But I also miss a lot when I do. I told you and told you." The lines on her face deepened and her features crumpled. "No one understands."

1

"Tell me again," I said. (Be patient. She's your Mom.)

"My hearing aid brings your voice closer, but it also brings me the sound of the faucet drip in the kitchen, fifteen feet away, the whistle of the teakettle, the bubbling of the coffee percolator, even the bark of the neighbor's dog down the block. How would *you* like it if you had to listen to all that hullabaloo?"

"Oh, come on, Ma. You're exaggerating."

She chuckled. "Well, maybe a little. But I have to, because nobody wants to believe me. And they shout. How would you like it if people always shouted at you? It makes me feel I've done something wrong."

"I wasn't shouting. I was just raising my voice."

"Then try to raise it more gently, like this." With a simpering expression and a childlike lilt in her voice, she repeated, word for word, my question to her ten minutes earlier. "Do you need anything from the store, Mom? I'm going shopping." We both laughed at her mimicry.

"So you did hear me after all."

"Finally."

"What do you mean, 'finally'? Why didn't you answer right away?"

"It takes time to answer—not exactly that—it takes time for my hearing to get up there, in my head. You should wait for my brain to process what you've said."

With the first glimmer of insight I pursued this scoop.

"How much time?"

"A few seconds, perhaps."

"But that's not a lot," I said, feeling contrite.

"Is that so? Well, people don't wait for me to catch up. Let me tell you something that I read. On the average a speaker rattles off at least ten words in a second. That means if you go on talking for five seconds it amounts to about fifty words I've lost. Do you know what that means?"

I calculated rapidly, remembering that after asking my question I had quickly explained when and why I was about to leave home.

"You see?" she said triumphantly. "You kept on talking and in my head I was racing to catch up. I could have made it, with three extra seconds to go on, but you went right ahead and shouted at me that—"

"I *didn't* shout."

"Yes, you did. You shouted something about why I wasn't wearing my hearing aid."

"I wasn't shouting at *you*, Mom. I was just making sure you'd hear me. I'm sorry."

"It's okay," she said and rewarded me with a kiss.

ONE

Sound and Fury

My friends used to call me a Yoga buff. The word "Yoga" printed on a poster tacked to an electric pole or a tree trunk sent a thrill of anticipation through me. I would interrupt any conversation with a walking companion and stop to read the date and place at which the class was to take place. During my field trips, as I traveled to attend a conference, or stayed at a vacation resort, I would check in at a Yoga center for a relaxing retreat.

This habit led me to a one-time Yoga session in, of all places, the gymnasium of a high school on the Upper West Side of New York City. I was a stranger to my classmates, and in fact most of them did not know each other. We at once formed a fraternity, bound by the earnestness of the instructor and the enticing nature of Hatha Yoga itself.

We were lying on our own separate bath towels covering the hard acrylic polish of the gym floor, chests arched in the Classic Plough Yoga posture. I was lost in spiritual retreat, my body firmly arched with my head back, pressing against the rigid floor. I must have been meditating with my eyes closed for three or four minutes when I felt a gentle tap on one leg. My back flattened as I opened my eyes and was startled to see a strange expression, slightly amused, on the face of the instructor, who was squatting on his haunches, motioning me to rise. All around me I could see some thirty or forty pairs of legs supporting bodies fully upright. Quickly I pulled myself up to join the rest of the class, all of whom seemed to be staring at me, looking as puzzled as I felt. Why was everybody standing? Or rather, why was I not?

Class continued in a few seconds. It was by now obvious to me that I, alone, had not heard the leader's instruction for us to rise and assume an upright Yoga posture. When did so much happen? How long had I been lying prone, like a stray mute who had wandered into this crowd by mistake? Nobody explained what had occurred, but suddenly I *knew*. During the next series of exercises I found myself straining to hear the instructions. Finally, I caught on to a procedure that was to become a familiar device. I began watching my closest neighbor in the class for cues. I was desperate to avoid an embarrassing slip again, lest I be regarded as some sort of weirdo. How were my classmates to know, as I had realized at once, that I had simply not heard our teacher's instructions and that, with my eyes partly closed or focused on the ceiling, my hearing had not had the customary help of sight?

What hurt most was that I seemed to have been the *only one* in the whole crowd to have missed the instructor's words. A flutter of fear went through my veins as I registered a warning about what was likely to happen next time—or someday. I could not recall having failed on any previous occasion to hear what everyone else around me heard. Little did I know that to those who knew me well, who communicated with me daily, my failure to hear was common knowledge. It's one of those things, like halitosis, that your best friends don't like to tell you. And how else would you know, if family and friends willingly accommodated your handicap by repeating what they had said or asked or just dropped the subject? Ah, the patience and kindness that grace our days, of which we are so unaware that we fail to add these blessings to those we recount in our prayers!

This single incident stands out as a time when my private inner life abruptly changed. Never again would I remain unfazed when I needed to ask, "What did you say?" Whenever I failed to hear, I remembered the embarrassing scene in the gym. Something was wrong with me— something I dared not tell—so that I was powerless to deal with it. I learned to steel myself to keep straining with the strictest attention in any noisy environment where I knew I would suffer failure to catch on. It happened often when everybody started to laugh. I learned to laugh along while my heart missed a beat. If the ensuing conversation dealt with the joke, I remained in a rigid state of suspense until the joke had been fully savored and dismissed.

All of us carry about a stream of subconscious thoughts, as Freud made clear when he described the method of deep analysis which he pioneered. We have learned that the minutest details of a lifetime's experiences remain stored in our brain, images that record our past and return when provoked by something that has occurred in a conscious state. Each fleeting image bears a message, but usually we deem such memories whimsical and bed them down again with careless disregard. Occasionally, however, an image demands attention because it bears a more significant relation to the drift of our present awareness, something that has become suddenly important.

I had this experience after I began to suspect that my hearing was changing. The memory of one long-forgotten situation returned abruptly. In my mind's eye I saw the intent, listening stance of a valued colleague who, for all the years we worked together, carried about his neck a little black box that he fingered continuously during a conversation. He manipulated the switches on this gadget more actively at meetings and during long conference sessions. He was using a hearing aid most common at that time. All of us at the office valued the contribution that "Tom" made. He had a unique, sweeping kind of intellect that could analyze in a few minutes the substance of a discussion, distill it, and offer a series of suggestions that helped to establish agreement and productive conclusions. But time took its toll. His fumbling with the switches on his black box seemed to become more and more agitated, and occasionally his failure to catch the gist of the conversation was reflected in an irrelevant response or sheer silence. Gradually we ceased to pay attention to Tom; it was so much easier to converse with people who didn't slow us up.

When Tom retired I had no contact with him for several years until we met on the subway platform just below Carnegie Hall in New York City, where I had gone to attend a concert of the Boston Symphony Orchestra. I assumed, correctly, that he had attended the same concert; we both made a hasty stab at a few words that were pretty much obliterated by the thunder and rumble of the noisy subway trains passing on both the uptown side and the downtown side of the platform. We gave up trying to talk and merely waved good-bye to each other as we boarded our separate trains. I was sorry that our meeting was over so soon, but I assumed that Tom was anxious to catch the last commuter train to his suburban home, and I made a hasty judgment that it was wise to end this sudden reunion. (How I wish I could do this whole scene all over again today!) I was happy to learn that he was still able to hear enough to enjoy a performance of this splendid symphony. I have since learned that hearing-impaired people usually retain enough ability to reap the pleasure of music for most of their lives, especially through the rhythmic vibrations and changing sound frequencies, in spite of the fading of the senses.

I had no contact with Tom for about five years after he retired. We were both isolated in our separate suburbs many miles apart. I was delighted, therefore, to see him at an office reunion of retired staff. We chose seats at the same table for the luncheon session. During this two-hour period the schedule called for one or two speakers from the dais, and time remained for table discussion. Tom's movements were slow and careful as he seated me ceremoniously beside him—more gentle, almost romantic, as I certainly did not remember him, in his eagerness to revive our friendship. His complexion was pale, not as I remembered it, the skin softly sagging, but his eyes still twinkled with the lively intelligence and the joy we both felt, anticipating a closing of the gap of mutual retirement. Naively, I had expected to resume conversing with Tom at about the place where we had left off many years ago. Alas, that was not to be.

The black box was still in place on his chest, his fingers still played around with the gadget, but it seemed to me a dead object, judging by the progress of our conversation. I tried several subjects, making an effort to speak distinctly. I know, now, as I did not realize at the time, that for a hearing-impaired person about the worst place to attempt a private tête-a-tête is a room full of other people who are also engaged in conversation with each other. The situation worsens when plates are rattling and waiters are stomping (or so it seems), their steps pounding beneath one's ears as they lug trays laden with dishes. Tom never once succeeded in catching the gist of my conversation. He seemed simply to wait until I stopped. Then he quickly seized his opportunity to pick up where he had left off.

As an attempt to touch bases in friendly exchange, this reunion was for me a total disaster. Little by little I gave up trying to reach Tom and gave him the floor altogether. (I have only recently learned that one of the strategies of a partially deaf person may be to keep talking excessively in order to avoid those terrible lapses in communication when a partner who has lost the drift of a conversation that is full of seemingly irrelevant information stops talking altogether.) He seemed to be aware that my attention was wandering, but he continued to rattle on in an almost frantic effort to reengage my interest. Finally his attenuated monologue became actually boring, and I lost the thread of the story, if there was one, that he was telling. Guiltily I looked forward to the end of the luncheon session and my chance to escape. I was simply worn out! The guilt mounted as the day wore on, when I noticed that others were also avoiding Tom; it becomes difficult to establish a personal reunion with someone who seems only remotely aware of what is going on. The rest of us, the lucky ones, were coasting along on a journey of pleasant memories. For a few days after Tom and I parted I was haunted by the pleading look on his face as I offered my hand to bid him good-bye.

After my experience in the gym, the memory of this encounter, which had receded over the years, loomed ominously large, and I vividly recalled my original remorse. I tried to forget the image, but it would not go away. I found myself unable to ignore my apprehension. Was this to be my fate as well?

Still another image emerged, triggered by the memory of Tom. This one went much further back, to the time when I was a college freshman. Mrs. H., a sweet little old lady who lived with her daughter and husband had invited me to spend a week in their home while I was recuperating from a hospital stay. I was cared for by their friendly housekeeper, who had formerly worked as a practical nurse. For company while my hosts were away at work I had, apart from the housekeeper, only the eighty-year-old mother, who kept to the privacy of her room most of the day. We came together at mealtimes. She too had one of those little black boxes dangling from a leather band around her neck, but it seemed useless, as she never fingered the switches. She was almost totally deaf; perhaps some vibration through the box alerted her to signals such as a doorbell, or a telephone, so that she could understand the housekeeper's movements.

Otherwise it served only to inform me of the stark reality of her impairment.

Her conversation was so fragmented as to be disquieting. She spoke in a very low voice, possibly not realizing how low, and although my hearing had not then begun to deteriorate, listening was tiring. It was even worse to try to make her understand my voice, deliberately raised until it was too loud. My ridiculously exaggerated lip movements were the more confusing because they did not match my gestures. I was disappointed and even ashamed of my failure to succeed in communicating, for this dear woman was an intelligent, cultured person who, I knew, had much to share. Whenever she left her room, she clutched a book, always a classic, by such authors as Thackeray, Trollope, and—since she had had a French education—Flaubert in the original French, which she held out for me to see.

I felt sad for her, but also I felt lonely, and the frustration caused by my abortive attempts to fill the hours of each quiet day made me wish for the week to end. Since communication broke down when it was attempted on an intellectual level, she tried shifting to simpler subjects. Pointing almost apologetically to the leftover half of a slice of toast, she explained that the housekeeper knew this was to be served to her during lunch. She had an almost continual smile suggestive of gentle resignation. She seemed eons removed from the excitement of my own active life. The ravages of age and affliction were only momentarily evident on her face. The pale cheeks were crepey. Dry strands of white hair clung in thin wisps across her ear lobes. Even in my convalescent state it seemed that my youthful buoyancy must be an affront to this feeble woman silenced and isolated by her impairment. I felt little kinship with her as I listened.

As I recall these two scenes, dredged up from a buried past and infused with new significance, I try to imagine a better more useful way in which we might have related to each other. My failure at the time seems callous, in the light of my present understanding of how the lucky ones, who can hear, who live in the "real" world, can reduce the sense of alienation that pervades our other world—the world of those who can't hear. The invisible handicap has become visible in my case as I've conscientiously strived to be open about it. I am learning to connect and to bridge the gap of understanding in my own case. I hope that this book will further that mission.

I think of the many things that Tom and I could have talked about to our mutual pleasure. For one thing, I would, today, have referred openly to his hearing problem and asked how he was managing. Perhaps I would have let him know with gestures toward my ear, how I, and anyone, may have frequent lapses in hearing, so that his dysfunction seemed less of a personal affliction. I might have asked him whether I was speaking too fast, or too loudly. All this I could accomplish, I'm sure, with gestures.

In the case of Mrs. H., the whole scene becomes more elaborate as I look back. Two weeks after the visit, I returned to college and a course on the contemporary American novel. During class, I recalled that I had noticed on Mrs. H.'s bookshelf a copy of Theodore Dreiser's *An American Tragedy* and several books by Sinclair Lewis, all examples of the contemporary American novel at that time, which we were discussing in class. I kept wondering how I could have approached her on this subject. After all, when I traveled through Europe I was often able to manage to communicate with people who spoke a different language. Why couldn't I have stimulated this withdrawn person to discuss the books she was reading? Why didn't I remove the Dreiser book, or a Lewis book, from the shelves and show her passages that I especially liked? Why didn't I take Flaubert's *Madame Bo-*

vary when she held it out to me, and speak to her of the passages that seemed to find an echo in the work of American novelists?

The three situations I've revived in such detail reflect with remarkable accuracy three stages that hearing-impaired people generally experience. It is testimony to the mysterious logic of the subconscious that I recalled these three scenes not chronologically but in the same sequence that marks the gradual progress of the dread handicap.

The first episode, involving my embarrassment in the gym, describes the initial stage of *denial*, when the afflicted person responds to the ominous warning signs by trying to avoid their significance and to keep the secret from leaking. Thus begins the long process of denial, first to oneself, and later to more and more people who dare to suggest that you have obviously failed to hear them.

Tom's behavior, excessive talking, follows years of failed communication, when one keeps making irrelevant responses, interrupts speakers without having heard them, and jumps in with comments on an entirely different subject—thus destroying the conversation, which may then come to an abrupt halt. Ultimately the disappointed listeners tend to ignore and to override the interruptions. Often they merely leave the floor to the interrupter, who may continue with a monologue as they secretly resolve to avoid him or her in the future. In the effort to remain involved, to hold the attention of the group, the hearing-impaired person has lost them. Tom was actually pleading, ''Listen to me. I'm still here. Don't cut me off.'' But nobody cares. The second stage, then, is the *breakdown of communication*.

Ultimately Tom feels forgotten and lonely. He contributes to his own ostracism when participation becomes an overwhelming strain and the world's indifference leaves him weary and discouraged. He chooses solitude to revive his energy. In the third stage, he gradually resorts more and more often to *withdrawal* for release, becoming less and less communicative. Those who don't know that he has a hearing problem regard his behavior as "peculiar," that of a recluse, an oddball, someone not quite with it—so that he seems to be the kind of person to be avoided.

When his impairment is so far advanced that it is no longer invisible, he becomes like all other handicapped people. He is now doubly isolated because most people tend to keep their distance from people who are seriously disabled and therefore "different." For him society has shaped itself into two separate worlds—the world of the normal people and the "other" world of the handicapped. Never again will he forget that he has been consigned to the latter.

About five years after the incident in the gymnasium I went out for a stroll in a city where I had just registered at a hotel for a week-long business meeting. I was orienting myself as I usually did after unpacking. I noticed the sign on a storefront: FREE HEARING TEST. I had seen such free tests advertised many times much closer to home, not only on storefronts, but in newspaper ads, in magazines, and on television. Not for me, I told myself once again. I was not consciously oppressed by an occasional failure to hear.

My acceptance of the inconvenience stemmed partly from a workshop I had attended on active listening. The psychologist who addressed us was armed with a portfolio of research material on the techniques of listening and the characteristics of a good listener. He began by citing some startling information. Studies of listening quality have shown that all of us hear only about 40 percent of the words that are spoken to us during normal conversation. Only rarely does a person listen so closely as to absorb most of the words spoken. It does happen occasionally, for example, when a student is intent on making notes at a class lecture or when a lawyer is engrossed in gathering material for rebuttal during a court proceeding. Otherwise we are able to understand the entire word if we have missed several syllables. This shorthand style of listening is honed by years of practice. Then, as a bonus, there is the speaker's tendency to repeat. (No longer do I complain "She talks too much" when a friend lingers repetitively over a story.) How many times have you been distracted during a conversation and yet remained fully capable of resuming listening without having lost the thread? Listening, according to the workshop leader, covers a wide range of possibilities. Fortunately, even a person with a slight hearing defect can get by for years because we've all had lifelong practice in making the most of fragmented hearing.

The original purpose of the workshop was to penetrate the subject much further, however. It was to demonstrate the power of creative listening, when a level of understanding is reached that shatters the wall of superficial attention with empathy and caring. Such listening is an act of love, a spiritual adventure by which we touch each other more richly in human encounter. I was to learn years later how much more incisive my listening had become because of the habit formed of necessity. I have learned to pay the closest attention to the speaker—not only to the sound of words, but to gestures, facial expression, tone, pitch, inflection, and emotional timbre. Later in this book I will enlarge on other positive aspects of handicaps.

I have often had occasion to cite these and other facts presented during the workshop. Occasionally I surprise and amuse people by quoting the psychologist's opening remarks. But the impact of his message served to reassure me that I was not facing imminent disaster when I happened to miss a few words or even a whole sentence; I was at such times *just like everybody else*. I was still effective in my work, even when I had to conduct interviews. Often I conducted the interview on the telephone and recorded it on tape to be reviewed later.

The free hearing test caught my attention because of the anonymity I would enjoy in a city 200 miles from where I lived or worked. Most people, I gather, have at some time been curious about how well they can hear, which is probably why the free hearing test offer is used so commonly as a come-on. Why not take the plunge, I thought, and find out at last? No one back home need know.

I entered a small room, barely but neatly furnished, where an alert receptionist greeted me and directed me to another room. A man approached me, introduced himself, and with a friendly handshake immediately came to the point. Had I ever had a hearing test? Why did I want one now? "It's a good idea," he agreed, to determine my hearing level, and he was sure he could help me do that. He pointed to a window in the wall of this little room and explained that he would be listening to me from the other side, using instruments to record my performance, while I used a device inserted first in one ear and then in the other.

I confessed (absurdly) that I was not a local resident, that I was actually not prepared to make any serious decisions about my hearing. "Perhaps I shouldn't have come in," I said, feeling a little ashamed that I had.

"Never mind," he protested, although his smile was slightly less cordial. I could hardly fault him for rushing me through the examination. It was a simple procedure, and I responded so easily that I was sure I was passing that examination with very high marks. The test was finished in less than ten minutes. It took about as much time as stopping at a minimart to pick up a loaf of bread. The examiner returned to the room, where I still had paraphernalia attached to my ears.

"Your hearing is normal for the present," he reported, as he scanned a small slip of paper that had been marked to show the sum of my responses on a graph. "You might get yourself tested again in a year or two." Sweet words—or were they?

This verdict should have been a welcome relief but unsurprisingly was not. I suppose a psychologist would easily have understood why I submitted to a test after first warning the examiner that I was a very bad risk as a potential customer. The significance of my ambivalence was not lost on me either, and I have gone into all the details of this event because it illustrates exactly how someone with my concern will persist in denial.

Before departing, I ventured to raise a question that I knew would otherwise haunt me thereafter.

"Then why is it that in the theater, or at a large meeting, I often miss something that's being said?"

"You'd be surprised," he said, with a little chuckle, "how many other people there are who are also missing dialogue. They just don't tell you. Why should they? Do you tell them?"

That piece of information, given its source, filled me with as much joy as a gift of roses, and I left his little office in a state of delicious euphoria. But the apprehension I had suffered for years inevitably returned, and I decided I would test out his comment the next time I found myself embarrassed when I laughed like everyone else at something I had not actually heard in the theater.

"What did he say?" I asked the woman seated on my right.

She shrugged. "I didn't really hear," she said.

I turned to the young man on my left "What was that all about?" I asked. With a gesture of hands, he answered, "I don't know, but it looked pretty funny."

The test and the ensuing incident at the theater, innocuous on the surface, had the effect of further delaying any effort on my part to face the obvious for a full six years! I was still focused comfortably on my busy, fulfilling life and could ignore negative intrusions. I was engrossed in my career as an editor and free-lance writer, fortunate in my marriage, and pleased and proud of my family life at home. I had passed successfully through my midlife crisis and arose each morning ready for the adventure of a new day.

I am amazed now at how well I was able to sustain the fantasy while a series of events continued to imperil my serenity. Perhaps self-delusion, largely subconscious, is a gift, a valuable form of protection. It becomes aberrant, however, when a problem exists that cannot be ignored. A time came when my family began to pay part of the price for my refusal to face reality. I was using all my energy in futile denial. Six years later an audiologist was to inform me, "Your procrastination was a normal reaction. In fact, you were even one year ahead. On average, a person waits seven years before taking action *after* he has already decided 'to do something about my hearing'!"

During those six years I kept learning more tricks to sustain the illusion. My behavior changed in subtle ways. My defenses shrouded me like a cocoon. I was always searching for a key to the half-heard words of a speaker. I had to pretend, often to lie. ("Sorry, I misunderstood you on the telephone. A noisy truck was just passing by outside.") When I missed part of a question, I took chances by nodding or smiling. Sometimes, mercifully, the ploy worked or seemed to (I was never sure). I watched people closely for clues as to what was being said in order to avoid asking them to repeat. I learned to moderate my penetrating stare, hoping that people might simply feel flattered by my respectful attentiveness. I complained frequently about the acoustics in a large room, at conferences, even in someone's home when a television emitted a jumble of confusing sounds.

In a restaurant, harassed by the noise, I struggled to

17

understand when a waiter or my companions were making suggestions about what to order, after I explained that I didn't like fried foods or things smothered in sauce. I have never forgotten, nor have the other diners at my table, when two waiters in starched white caps appeared balancing a huge oval-shaped platter. It was tented with a covering of searing foil. One waiter pierced the cover and displayed a slippery silver coil. It was steamed eel! Under the foil was an assortment of more edible seafood, while I reached with clumsy fumbling, noting that nothing was fried or covered in sauce.

I endured comments such as the following, pretending I didn't mind:

"The trouble with you is, you don't listen."

"Let's not sit so close to the music. After all, this isn't a rock and roll concert."

"But I just *said* that—only a minute ago!"

"Don't be so fussy about where the hostess places us. It's embarrassing." (I couldn't make a joke out of that one.)

I felt cut off from the normal world by such ordinary remarks. A wall was rising between the two worlds I straddled. Occasionally I imagined people were trying to distance themselves from me because my presence was such an inconvenience. They couldn't know how that hurt. I had no right to tell them.

Meeting people for the first time was a hazard. Soon I developed a knack for catching a person's name but it didn't always work. One such conversation when my maneuver bombed went something like this:

"Sorry. I didn't catch your name."

The name is repeated.

"I beg your pardon. How do you spell it?"

"Spell it??? SMITH. Smith."

"Oh! [smile] Just kidding."

In fact, the slight sound of the consonant *s* becomes very confusing for a person with presbycusis, the type of hearing loss that most often afflicts the elderly. It comes off too much like *f*, *v*, or *sh*. The same is true of the sound of *th*. So an introduction to a Smith can be ominous as the beginning of a new acquaintance. Once when I asked a young woman to repeat her first name, she did so and added "with a C, not a K." With this extra clue I guessed that she was saying "Catherine." Correct! I felt as if I had just won a spelling bee.

Family members enjoy the freedom to criticize each other (or what's a family for?). But I was the beneficiary of rather a lot of privileged candor. I tried to avoid acknowledging why I hadn't heard the visitor knocking at the door, the telephone ringing in the next room. I was told that someone upstairs who asked me to "turn down the television for God's sake" wasn't yelling at me. My husband had to remind me that the timer on the stove was buzzing ("Didn't you hear it?"), that I had left the faucet dripping, that a squawk from the microwave had reached his desk in the study.

He did it by teasing. "You're not getting *that* old."

"Of course not, but hang in there. It's coming."

Such banter, in the context of our enduring relationship, served to assuage my early discomfort. Thus far I had been able to tolerate the deprecatory comments with which we played our roles as loyal conspirators in a long and happy companionship. When eventually the pleasantries carried a faint sting on both sides, I began to feel undeservedly guilty. How was I to dodge the warning signs without admitting that I was having trouble with my hearing? Often I came near to confessing and quickly backed down. I know now that I was actually afraid (of what?) and was angry that I was afraid.

The most pervasive fear concerned the ring of the telephone, a sound that all my life had filled me with anticipation. I had always rushed to answer, ready for a warm human encounter. My daughter had a sweet practice of reaching for the phone to call me whenever something pleasant occurred. I loved such surprises. Often a colleague called with some helpful information for the article I was writing at the office. Now the first ring of the phone gave me palpitations. Every muscle tensed. I began to keep notes in my head of which caller had the kind of voice that projected poorly. I closed windows, turned down the heat under a bubbling percolator, and prayed that the caller would be someone I could hear easily, preferably a woman with the high-pitched voice that projected well for my particular kind of impairment. What would I do if the caller was a rapid speaker, or shouted, or mumbled, or whose voice sounded mushy and seemed to get smothered in telephone lines? How many times did I dare ask the caller to repeat a sentence, without arousing impatience or puzzlement or eliciting the abrupt response "see you—good-bye" and hanging up? Sometimes, from necessity, I called on anyone in the room or nearby, to record an important message accurately, although I regretted the loss of privacy and independence. I hated feeling childish and humiliated.

Most upsetting was my inability to carry on a cozy conversation with my daughter. All my family called Susan a "miracle baby" because thirteen years had passed before we were blessed with the arrival of our first and only child. After my prayers were answered, there was never a moment in the years of her growing up when her voice failed to resonate to the "miracle" of her presence. I always looked forward to our telephone conversations. Susan is young and a fast talker. The words pour forth with racing speed, full of enthusiasm. "I've only got a minute," she would warn me and then stay on the phone for ten.

Now when I picked up the receiver and heard my daughter's cheery "Hi, Mom," the lyrical quality of her voice brought a nervous quiver to my ears. I couldn't keep up with her pace and missed half of what she was saying. Sooner or later she would stop her chatter and ask a question. That habit floored me. Often I didn't know what she had been telling me. After a strange pause she would say, "Didn't you hear me?" I hesitated to ask her to rephrase her question when I had already made a few silly mistakes that she had corrected with a giggle. One day she began to resort to a new strategy. After I had answered and had given her some news, she would say, "Let me talk to Dad." After Lou had hung up, I would have to make do with a man's laconic summary, devoid of the gossipy details that make talk between women such fun. Almost always Susan had some important matter she needed to discuss and wanted the more seasoned and logical opinion she expected from her father. I knew it was childish to feel rejection. But like a six-year-old, I did.

Eventually I too adopted a similar strategy and asked the caller to turn the telephone over to someone else. I did so particularly when the caller's voice was pitched in the low-frequency area. In music it would be characterized as a bass sound. In this area I have my greatest difficulty. The voice in question is usually a man's. When the husband of one of my friends called I cut the conversation short, hoping he would forgive my abrupt dispatch of business. Oddly, this won me kudos with him. "What I like about your telephone calls, Charlotte, is that you make them short. You deal with the essentials and say goodbye."

Many of the men who call are middle-aged workmen who need some particular information: the plumber, the electrician, the telephone repairmen, the insurance man. When Lou is home I immediately transfer the receiver to him and let him deal with the caller. The age of the caller makes a difference too. Unlike members of Susan's high-powered generation, older people speak more slowly. They pause often, hesitate, and repeat. This behavior allows more time for a message to travel along the hearing nerve to the brain, where comprehension results, the final goal of a complicated journey. The journey begins in the outer ear, goes through the ear canal to the eardrum, to the three tiny bones in the middle ear, to the nerve endings in the cochlea of the inner ear that direct the hearing nerve to the brain. Imagine how I shuddered when a fast talker plunged into his message on the telephone. When I was alone at home I felt bereft.

Not everyone appreciated my abbreviated phone calls. Many people have told me that I hung up while they were still talking! To them it seemed funny—but not to me. Such news caused a heaviness in my chest that lasted for hours. This tendency to succumb to the negative aspects is familiar to audiologists, who know that the hearing-impaired person begins to develop symptoms of paranoia. The tendency is especially pronounced when there is some basis for suspicion, as a psychologist would confirm. I came to recognize "the look" when two people who had witnessed a blunder in my response turned to each other with poker faces. If there was laughter in the room when I hadn't heard the joke, or if it came too soon for my slower hearing mechanism to register the sound in my brain, I was uncomfortable. Why was everybody laughing? Were they laughing at me? Had I said something stupid? Anyone with normal hearing who had missed the point of a joke might calmly request that it be repeated, but I didn't dare. I wouldn't risk letting other people know of my hearing loss.

Some consequences of my failure to understand a message are etched in my memory forever. Once I waited two hours for my dinner guest in the lobby of a restaurant, frequently checking at the bar, hoping that she would eventually arrive. The occasion was a farewell dinner before she moved to a distant state. We had arranged the date over the phone. Several times I ventured away from the spot where I was waiting, to make phone calls, but no one answered at her home. I kept dashing in and out of the lobby to speak to managers and hostesses of three nearby restaurants, leaving a message. Finally, at about ten o'clock I left for home, limp and worried. As I sat chewing on a rubbery, tasteless cheese sandwich, the phone rang and an agitated voice asked,

"Where have you been?"

"Waiting—at the restaurant. What happened?"

"I just got home. You weren't there. Are you O.K.?"

She had been waiting at the Homestead. I was standing outside a place some twenty blocks north, under a sign that read "Homestyle Restaurant." I hadn't heard the second part of the name when we spoke on the phone about the appointment. She apologized for the misunderstanding, feeling less vulnerable. I lacked the courage to explain that it was my error, for the admission might reveal that I was hard of hearing, but my cowardice damaged my self-respect.

More than ten years have passed. On my dresser there is a little box of Réplique perfume—a gift from this friend, lost to me since the day of an aborted farewell. She had brought it to me after one of her trips abroad, knowing it was my favorite perfume. I have never used it; it sits there, keeping me forever attached to the sweet, sad memory of a cherished friendship.

Thereafter I established a procedure in making appointments. I learned to repeat the date, time, and place, to spell out key words of directions, and to listen closely when the speaker confirmed the information. I was honing my skill in listening and double-checking, a newfound ability that I would someday count among my blessings, when I had made peace with destiny.

During over twenty years while I was a director on the national staff of the YMCAs, I developed elaborate coping mechanisms to swim with the tide of a hearing decline. I used my wiles during staff meetings, week-long seminars, and occasional retreats at a conference center in a country setting. As editor of the national YMCA publication mailed out to the professional staffs of some 1,800 YMCAs in the United States and in thirteen foreign countries, I needed to keep track of the most significant activities in the local Ys and to report the social trends that Y directors should heed as they developed their community service programs. The meetings with national directors who had been traveling widely were a source of much information. The portfolios of these national directors covered distinct areas: physical education, young adult, older adult, camping, sports, teenagers, middle childhood, preschool, religion, and culture. My listening skills had become razor sharp; my curiosity was a source of amusement to my colleagues.

"Watch out for Charlotte. She won't miss a trick," a colleague warned. I hounded the directors with questions to fill any gaps in their reporting. My pen scratched continuously. I was alive with the excitement of new data, with sudden inspiration about how to apply, implement, and draw inferences as I identified connections with similar activities in other organizations. To be prevented from reaching my objective because of a gradual loss of hearing would be punishment indeed.

I had worked with most of the men and one or two other women on the staff for many years and enjoyed the camaraderie. Because of our full business portfolios, get-togethers gave us all a chance to touch base, even with a demanding agenda. I cherished the opportunity at the opening of a meeting when each of us had a scheduled time to speak of our progress or lack of progress, our triumphs, our disappointments, and our hopes for the coming months. This time of sharing set the tone that made it possible to effect compromises, accept our differences, and reach consensus without conflict.

I began to be wary of differences in the way individuals projected their voices. One or two spoke very softly. I tried to select a seat near them. One spoke with lips almost closed. This habit presented the worst problem. One had a habit of dropping his voice on the final words of a sentence so low that I sometimes lost the gist of the message. The change in my sound reception was gradual and for perhaps three years did not diminish my effectiveness and participation. I knew when I needed to listen very sharply. I reached meetings early and observed where others chose their seats, then chose mine very carefully so as to be closest to people whose speech gave me trouble. I practiced so that I could accommodate unusual speech habits. I remember that one person lowered his head and shuffled papers at the beginning of his talk. Ultimately all of my maneuvers were still not sufficient to bail me out. I had to strain increasingly to catch a crucial phrase. When I missed, I stiffened so as not to miss the main point of the ensuing discussion. Occasionally I did ask for clarification, but I was careful not to overdo it. My technique was to make some slight gesture to a colleague, who would whisper a few words that put me back on track. I have never overcome the feeling of humiliation I suffered when a vote was being taken on whether or not we should postpone the next meeting until after the Christmas and New Year's holidays. Innocently, unaware of what was going on, I interrupted the voting by protesting that it would be a mistake to stay on schedule for our next meeting. "Why not," I suggested, "skip the next meeting because of the holidays?"

"That's just what we're voting on," said my neighbor. "Most of us agree. How about you?"

The chairman registered my vote without comment. No

one else commented either. I was on fire with humiliation. Had I appeared to be stupid? I scanned the faces around the table, looking for clues to their reaction. I hoped they assumed I had been distracted by some private concern. Bravely I smiled a self-deprecating smile, thus granting others the freedom to smile too. (They didn't.) I might have forgotten the incident if it had occurred just once. Such situations were repeated many times over the next few years, however, and contributed to my anxiety as I labored to concentrate on the proceedings.

I have discussed elsewhere the hazard of the telephone. Long distance calls presented a special problem in my work at the office, since they dealt more often with important affairs rather than casual social interchange. If my door was open, I was harassed by the bustle of the large outside staff. If I shut myself into the office I still had to adjust to the variation in voices on the phone. There were differences in mechanical transmission over the wires in different geographical locations or at different times of the day. I was subjected to noises in the room of the caller, as well as sudden outside noises at either end—trucks, traffic blasts, and ambulance sirens—and the tendency of people to shout to make themselves heard above the peripheral sound. I became tense instantly when answering a long distance call. I hated to keep asking the speaker to repeat, especially since I could not blame it on "a bad connection" if he was not having similar difficulty.

The memory still haunts me of the abrupt ending, with a long distance call, of a relationship that I had valued for more than twenty years. Hoby (a nickname I have changed here) was an office colleague for whom I had done some free-lance writing and editing. After he left our organization he phoned from his new location some 500 miles away. I could not recognize his voice or understand the name of the caller. For some reason my hearing was exceptionally poor that morning. It might have been the weather, or fatigue, or a bad phone connection, or perhaps Hoby was holding the receiver too far from his lips. The foggy sound that reached me seemed to be floating from a cloud a million miles away. He kept telling me his name, but I did not recognize it. He tried giving his name in full. He tried and tried. In my panic and frustration I could feel the decibels of my hearing loss rising alarmingly. Had I gone suddenly deaf? Eventually he hung up. I sat for a long time beside the phone and let the tears fall. I cried for all the hundreds of times I had struggled vainly to overcome my hidden impairment, for the embarrassment, the humiliation, the vexation, the fear. Later one night I woke to catch the end of a dream, a dream about Hoby, standing at a distance half hidden by a meadow of tall grass, and calling, calling. I had of course eventually identified him as the person who had given up trying to reach me on a long distance call. He will never know, unless he reads this someday, that I had not become senile or demented.

Being a mechanical moron, I resisted acquiring a tape recorder. Now I determined to acquire a good reliable Sony and practice using it. When I succeeded at last (tape recorders were crude equipment in those days) and taped my first long distance telephone interview, I felt I had found the secret passage out of a dark forest. Now I could check out whatever I had heard only in fragments and rejoice in the possibility of repetition. "Have no fear of repetition," advises the award-winning writer James Kirkpatrick. The same is true of the spoken word, as any successful lecturer has learned. A tape recorder throws a lifeline to a hard-of-hearing person. By using it, furthermore, I was able to dispense with the laborious distraction of notetaking.

One day I had a call from a couple of friends to suggest we join them in getting subscriptions to a series of Broadway plays. For years we had gone to the theater with them, and we readily consented. They suggested tickets for the first balcony beyond the mezzanine, our usual choice, matching our current budget. I would have liked to sit closer to the action but couldn't mention my reason.

The setting and lighting were beautiful for the first play. I was happy that the two women who sat in the row just below me seemed short, especially after they removed their hats. I listened comfortably to the opening lines during those magical first moments when a hushed audience watches for the promise of enchantment. Suddenly a door on the stage opened and a voice shattered the peaceful scene with a blast of angry sound. A man's voice uttered exaggerated protests, and the audience instantly laughed. Turning to my husband, I asked, "What was that all about?"

He stopped me with a gesture while trying at the same time not to miss the actor's next sentence. "Tell you later," he whispered, while I continued to fall further behind. (He never did tell me.) I struggled for the next five minutes before I was able to catch the thread of the plot. Another actor and his wife entered, carrying on an animated conversation, all the time stalking about noisily plumping up cushions, turning on lights, checking their faces in a mirror, and weaving a web of confusion that thwarted all my efforts at comprehension.

After I had grasped the plot, I was able to enjoy the play, although I was still losing quite a few lines. Fortunately conversation among performers often includes repetitive phrases for dramatic effect or for emphasis, so that it is not necessary to hear all that is said.

I have since learned (although I still forget at times) not to demand immediate help when I haven't heard a word. Sometimes comprehension, while the brain is processing the sound, takes a slight fraction longer for a hard-of-hearing person; if I wait, I may then "hear" the word. But even more important, there's an etiquette to be followed out of consideration for the person who endures the distraction of my behavior. At times I resign myself to remaining uninformed. Even my husband, who is my dearest friend in accommodating all my needs, could not always be patient with the jabs of my elbow against his ribs.

I awoke one morning feeling unaccountably exhilarated. Something had happened in my sleep, some dream lost to awareness on awakening. My eyes searched the familiar furnishings of my room, the family photographs on the dresser, the framed print we had brought back from Florence of St. Francis of Assisi feeding his birds, the plump down cushion I must have tossed to the floor during my sleep. Everything looked new and vivid, somehow more real, as though all the varied parts of my life had moved into place and had enabled me to become whole, fully in charge. For the first time I understood the phrase so often used by my teenage granddaughter and her friends: "She's got it all together." Lying there with my head comfortably pillowed on one arm, I felt alive and at peace. I knew at once that I was going to make an important decision. I would give up my futile role of deception; it wasn't working anyhow. I had had too many signs that my hearing loss was becoming more and more obvious.

To my surprise, in deciding to be open and break the silence I experienced a tremendous high. I could be as free as I wanted to be! I could admit that I hadn't heard, explain when my hearing failed, change my seat in any room, ask permission to turn up the television slightly, and casually say to the man who rang my doorbell, "I'm hard of hearing. Can you say that again, please?" I look back upon those six years when I wasted so much energy as more trying than any period thereafter. The battle to keep my hearing loss hidden had taken a greater toll than all that was to come later.

I began by telling my husband that I wanted to get my hearing tested. "It's about time," he said, keeping his voice low and calm. "I've been wondering how much longer you were going to wait." Next I told my daughter. "You really should," she said. "I'm glad you're going to do it." (Hers was a low-keyed response as she took the cue from her father.) Obviously, it was no secret to them! How many other people knew?

Characteristically, I turned my resolve into a research project. What leads should I follow to get professional guidance? Was there someone I knew who might help me? What questions should I be asking? I went first to the library to look up the literature on the subject of hearing.

TWO

Hearing and Hearing Loss

When I first began to study the technical material about the physiology of the ear I was so overwhelmed by its intricacy that I was tempted to give up. How fortunate that I persevered. I found myself intrigued, reverential, and determined to unravel the mumbo-jumbo of the technical treatises. As I read, it increasingly seemed to me that a divine Entity must be responsible for this miracle of engineering.

The problem of how we hear has been debated for hundreds of years. There are a number of theories, the four principal ones being the place theory, the frequency theory, the volley theory, and the traveling wave theory. All of these have their ardent supporters, and yet there is a great deal more that scientists have not yet been able to explain. Numerous descriptions appear in printed brochures, on posters, and in leaflets in doctors' waiting rooms. Some facts, however, are generally supported by theorists.

The external ear is relatively little involved in the hearing process. It consists of a flap of cartilage that is a neat and graceful boundary of the organ and also serves as a foundation for earrings. The lobe helps trap sound. Hard of hearing people in the earliest stage of loss often cup the palm of the hand behind the ear. This is an attempt to trap the vibrations of sound and to block off peripheral noise. The gesture helps only a little, as you will discover if you try it yourself. When Van Gogh, the eccentric artist, in his madness and frustration over a scorned love, cut off his ear, his sense of hearing did not diminish. When you were a child you may have gawked at an adult who could perform the trick of "wiggling" an external ear. Very few people can voluntarily move the muscles involved.

Within the ear, interconnected activities take place. Without your turning your head, you can locate sounds from behind you, from far away; your inner ear distinguishes a faint whisper, a remote hum. Each separate musical note, the thousands of musical sounds and combinations from every variety of musical instrument, are all distinguished by the ear. It learns to tune out sounds that are useless when we don't want them, for example, all the night sounds of birds and insects outside my window and of foliage rustling in the wind, to which I remain oblivious during sleep. Even now I can detect the smallest change in the sound of my husband's breathing since he developed a heart ailment. This noise penetrates so that I respond and awaken immediately.

Sound journeys from the outer ear through the middle ear and the inner ear with its nerve passages (see figure 1). These sections comprise a system of electronics as dense as the telephone system wired to serve a city with a population as large as that of Birmingham, Alabama. The ear canal permits sound waves to enter the ear. The canal narrows as it penetrates farther, causing sound waves to become louder as they approach the eardrum. The vibration of the thin-skinned eardrum transmits amplified sound to the middle ear's three conduction levers, described in almost all popular texts as the hammer (malleus), anvil (incus), and stirrup (stapes)—bones so tiny that they would all fit on the tip of your small finger. These levers, through mechanical energy, create waves which are transmitted to the inner ear's snail-

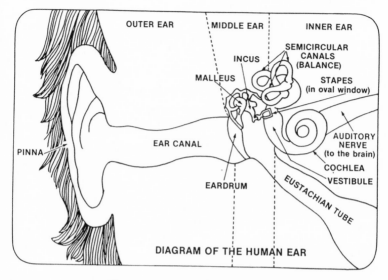

Figure 1. The structure of the ear.

shaped cochlea. Within the core of the cochlea microscopic hair cells are connected with some 27,000 to 30,000 nerve fibers in a fluid that is vibrated by the stirrings in the middle ear.* These tiny fibers are strong enough to support four tons of weight per square inch.

The pitch of sound caused by the frequency of the sound waves—vibrations per second—as the fluid travels through the hair cells ranges from high at the base of the cochlea to low at its apex. Electric currents are generated by the cochlea and travel through the nerve connections to the brain. The brain transforms the energy in the nerve connections to the intelligible sounds that we associate with comprehension. The human ear can distinguish and absorb more than 350,000 sounds, and from them the brain produces mean-

---

*The number of cells varies, depending on the source consulted. According to Newby and Popelka (1985), there is a ''single row of 3000 to 3500 inner hair cells and three or sometimes four rows of from 9000 to 12000 outer hair cells'' (p. 41). This estimate would indicate a total of between 27,000 and 47,000 cells.

ing. The outer and middle ear relays sound and creates its quantity (loudness). The pitch, whether high or low, is perceived by the inner ear.

In the course of a lifetime some of the hair cells wear out and die. There is never new growth, as there is with body hair or nails. As the hair cells continue to die, hearing is impaired because of the reduction in the connection between the middle ear and the inner ear. The steady death is directly associated with the process of aging, resulting in "presbycusis." As in my case, some time may elapse before you are aware of the loss.

The Otologist

When you first notice that you have been having difficulty hearing, you are not likely to ascribe the reason to a medical condition. Your doctor performing a routine checkup will always peer into your ears with a strong, concentrated light and will make no comment if nothing unusual is evident. Occasionally you may report some sensitivity, a feeling of stuffiness after swimming or during or after a drive through the country when you have ascended several thousand feet. Many people experience discomfort on a plane as it makes its descent for landing. Sometimes there's pain after a cold. If it lasts, your regular physician prescribes treatment for a temporary infection. Such common conditions correct themselves without causing you to seek help from an otologist, a physician specializing in medical treatment of the ears who is also known as an otolarynogologist, an otorhinolaryngologist, and an ear, nose, and throat man (ENT) because this branch of medicine encompasses all three organs.

If the pain persists, or if you have what's described as a "running ear," your private physician will suggest that you see the otologist, who diagnoses, treats, and performs surgery on ears. Many people who decide to do something about their hearing, however, bypass the visit to an otologist and go directly to an audiologist without realizing that hearing loss may be due to, or partly caused by, a medical problem which has gone undetected or ignored.

If you see an audiologist first, as most people tend to do, he will question you and look into your ears to determine whether there is any obvious indication of a complication requiring medical intervention. A ruling by the Food and Drug Administration, however, now requires "medical clearance" before a hearing aid is fitted because it is important to treat any physical problem first. If you are determined to avoid seeing an otologist, you may sign a waiver in the audiologist's office but it is not advisable to do so. The regulation in question reads:

> Federal law restricts the sale of hearing aids to those individuals who have obtained a medical evaluation from a licensed physician. Federal law permits a *fully informed adult* to sign a waiver statement declining the medical evaluation for religious or personal beliefs that preclude consultation with a physician. The exercise of such a waiver is not in your best health interest and its use is strongly discouraged.
>
> Following the medical evaluation the physician will give you a written statement that your hearing loss has been medically evaluated and that you may be considered a candidate for a hearing aid. The physician will refer you to an audiologist or a hearing aid dispenser, as appropriate, for a hearing aid evaluation. [*Federal Register*, vol. 42, no. 31, 1977; italics added]

If you are asked by an audiologist or hearing aid dealer to put your signature on a form, you should of course be sure to read it first. Even if you do sign a waiver and all obvious medical symptoms have been superficially checked, the audiologist will usually insist that you have an ear doctor clear out the wax in your ear, whether or not there is any substantial buildup, before making a mold for a hearing aid.

The otologist may simply find wax buildup but may detect early infection. An otological examination may uncover the first symptoms of hearing loss due to diseases such as muscular dystrophy or diabetes or evidence of metabolic disorders such as a high cholesterol level. Thus the otologist's routine physical examination may prove quite valuable. The many medical conditions that may involve hearing loss include otitis media, otosclerosis, tinnitus, Ménière's disease, tumors, and various neurological conditions.

Otitis media is the blockage of the oval window between the middle and inner ear due to immobility of the stapes bone that makes possible the transmission of sound. It may result from a cold or lung illness. There is a disturbance with the fluid that prevents the eardrum from working efficiently and may ultimately damage it. As a child you may have been told when you had a severe cold that you were blowing your nose too forcefully. It is difficult, especially for children, to refrain from doing so, but there is a danger that severe pressure from both nostrils will force mucus farther into the nasal passages, allowing bacteria to enter the ear. The result will be an inflammation or infection and often eventually a conductive hearing impairment. Most of us have had this kind of inflammation, however mild, at some time. In children it usually manifests itself as an earache, which is medicated and eventually heals itself. The proper way to blow the nose is to press lightly with the fingers on one nostril at a time without pinching the nostrils together. Try that on your red-nosed three-year-old!

Another common condition is "running ear," which may occur only occasionally and will heal automatically. When it keeps returning and becomes chronic it may result in hearing impairment.

Sources of other than respiratory infection include allergy, sinusitis, or blockage of the eustachian tube. If the infection persists in spite of recurrent treatment it may become chronic and cause hearing impairment. Breathing through the mouth in childhood is a signal of enlarged adenoids and/or allergy, which may result in hearing loss if the condition is not treated. The hearing loss may be too slight to be detected by an adult, especially because adults tend to raise their voices in talking to a child. Fortunately all children now have their hearing tested in school. Such tests may detect a hearing loss soon enough to help a child who does not always appear to be attentive. Afflicted children may legitimately protest, "But I didn't hear you."

The condition known as *otosclerosis* is hereditary and, though serious, can sometimes be corrected by microsurgery. It is a disease process that affects the bony capsule of the inner ear, turning the hard bone to a spongy substance. It is usually first noticed in young adulthood and progresses year by year. At first the problem involves the transmission of vibrations from the middle ear to the inner ear, but the disease may subsequently invade the inner ear, causing a sensorineural impairment. The loss may therefore involve both conductive hearing and nerve deafness. (I will discuss conductive and sensorineural types of loss shortly.) It is hereditary, is almost always accompanied by tinnitus, and usually progresses slowly to produce the hearing loss.

Tinnitus, a ringing or other noise in the ear, may signify a problem requiring attention beyond the scope of the audiologist's expertise, although perhaps half of those who complain of this disturbance visit an audiologist rather than first making an appointment with an otologist. It is caused by any one of a number of conditions that occur all along the passage through the ear, a buildup due to some poor function in the small bones, the muscles, or the eustachian tube. If it is high pitched, it may reflect some chemical disturbance between the cochlea and the brain. The sound is described in a variety of ways: as whistling, ringing, or humming, as a sound like that of steam escaping or even the roar of break-ers. If the sound is low-pitched, it may be an outer or middle ear affliction described as clicking, crackling, or rattling. Tin-nitus does not, of itself, cause deafness. Because it interferes with hearing, the audiologist can provide the mechanical means of treatment, mainly the hearing aid, but an otologist should be consulted first.

Anyone with normal hearing experiences tinnitus occa-sionally. For example, after a loud blast from a passing truck, we may continue to notice a noise in our head for some time. But the hard of hearing with tinnitus must endure these sounds constantly; in some cases the noise never stops. It is interesting that people with constant tinnitus often prefer a noisy room, where people tend to raise their voices loud enough to overcome the interference. Hearing-impaired in-dividuals in such cases benefit from the amplified voices of the speakers.

Another reported source of relief comes from staying within earshot of some other constant peripheral sound. A friend once told me she moved into an apartment close to a well-traveled highway, so that she is aware of the steady hum of traffic. The background sound, coming from several hundred yards away, drowns out the noise in her head. Because the noise comes from a distance, it seems less intru-sive and therefore actually affords some relief.

The treatment that this friend gave herself has since be-come standard: she provided a "masker" which would in-troduce an additional noise in the ear appropriately adjusted to her own tinnitus frequency. The audiologist can supply a mechanical masker for use during waking hours. It is not employed frequently, because tinnitus sufferers resist a de-vice which produces still more sounds with only limited relief.

Surprisingly often, people with tinnitus will tell me, "I've gotten used to it. . . . I just decided it was something

I'd have to learn to live with, and that's just what I've done." At least some degree of tinnitus is said to afflict as many as 38 million people in the United States, including some individuals with little or no other hearing loss. Sometimes conventional training in stress management, or other lessons in modifying one's behavior, relieves the tension.

This palliative does not apply generally to any other kind of hearing loss. In almost every case the hard of hearing must be resigned to live with the distress caused by the intrusion of peripheral sounds.

Menière's disease, which produces light-headedness, dizziness, nausea, and sometimes noises (tinnitus) in the ear, may be treated by drugs, although they do not always bring a permanent cure, and the end result may be permanent hearing loss. Jack Pulec, who has studied Menière's disease thoroughly, believes that the "causes unknown" include a viral infection, but he has been unable as yet to produce the statistical data to confirm this point (Pulec 1984:154–56).

The attacks may last a few minutes or several days and usually recur. Often they increase in severity causing some loss of hearing and sometimes total deafness. A patient who goes first to an audiologist will be referred immediately to an otologist, who is clinically trained to study and treat each patient medically. Tinnitus is often present where there is Menière's disease.

The otologist is able to detect other medical conditions that have resulted in hearing loss. A temporary blockage or spasm, for example, may interrupt the blood supply to the cochlea, so that tinnitus or sudden loss of hearing results. Perhaps the worst cause of hearing loss which a medical ear specialist may discover is a tumor at the base of the brain which can cause death unless microsurgery is performed.

The otologist looks for different reactions to drugs taken for medical conditions unrelated to the ear. Drugs may reduce the ability to hear in some people. This was especially true of quinine, which was formerly prescribed for malaria and sometimes for the common cold. Even aspirin taken in continuous and large doses may damage hearing in some people. Antibiotic drugs prescribed for too long a time may cause sensorineural loss, so most physicians carefully control the dosage and length of treatment.

The Audiologist

As I indicated earlier, people are often confused about the distinction between otology (a medical specialty) and audiology. The audiologist is professionally trained to evaluate hearing disabilities and to treat nonmedical aspects of impairment. This specialist has at least a master's degree in audiology and may also have earned a Ph.D. Each audiologist has worked with adults and children under supervision for at least 300 hours, has passed a national examination, and has spent one year of internship. Many states also require a license in audiology to practice (not to be confused with the license of a hearing aid dealer). The American Speech-Language-Hearing Association provides a certificate of clinical competence in audiology to qualified audiologists. (See appendix 4 for the address and phone number.) The audiologist identifies and assesses the degree of impairment and the type and variety of problems of communication that result; concentrates on ways to improve the client's hearing skills; determines whether a hearing aid will help; and offers the client an opportunity to select from a variety of aids, testing and measuring the improvement as each one is tried to identify the one best suited to the client. An audiologist also informs the client of other available listening devices and systems to help manage a hearing impairment and considers which, if any, other assistive devices to recommend.

Some audiologists, especially those in private practice, also sell hearing aids. If they do not, they will refer the client to a dealer and will later check the instrument selected. The audiologist will act as guide and supervisor while the client is using the new aid for a trial period, usually thirty days. All audiologists provide training in the use of hearing aids and follow-up consultation; the new user must learn to cope with the altered sounds that result when a mechanical instrument is used and must know how to care for the aid.

Audiologists are qualified to conduct workshops, lead support groups, train individuals and groups in speechreading (watching lips, faces, and body gestures of the speaker), and offer training in listening. Many are now offering aural rehabilitation, family counseling, workshops directed to employers and teachers, and consultation on ways of improving methods of communication and hearing conservation, training in the use of the telephone, and help with special telephone amplification.

Although some audiologists operate privately in an individual office, many are part of a team of associates to one of whom you may have been referred. If you see someone who is part of a team, you may also have contact with the other members on occasion, for example when the first arranges for consultation or when he (or she) is not available. Whenever you consult doctors or service specialists, of course, you should look for someone with whom you can work comfortably. Some flexibility on both sides may be called for; for example, when there's a temporary switch in the team. You will value the kind of sensitive support that a competent audiologist provides, as there will be a series of visits and continuous follow-up over the years to check changes in your hearing or to adjust the hearing instruments.

Many audiologists operate as members of a professional staff in a hearing center. They perform the standard services and support the other staff personnel who follow up with rehabilitation. Rehabilitative services at the center may include speechreading, training in listening and speaking, and counseling, especially during the period of orientation to a hearing aid. The center may have available for selection a number of aids produced by a variety of companies. The audiologist at the center assists the client in selecting the most suitable type of aid, a decision that depends on both the test results and the consultation. Years ago, it was hard to find a reliable hearing aid, and steep prices prompted unwary buyers to favor the aids that cost less. But hearing aids available for trial use in a center are safe today. The risks have been minimized because hearing aid parts are standardized and the aids are more reliable. A center will also check a client's purchase from a dealer who has agreed to the usual month's trial, to determine whether the model selected conforms with the center's evaluation and analysis of the individual's audiogram and consultation.

The National Association for Hearing and Speech Action has a help line that provides information about referrals to certified professional persons in your area who have met educational and clinical requirements. (See appendix 4 for the address and toll-free number.) Ask your physician to recommend an audiologist. You might also consult a friend or family member who has used an audiologist. Hospitals, universities, and colleges with speech, language, and hearing clinics are another source of referrals. Your telephone directory will list sources in public and private schools, industry, state and federal agencies with local offices, health departments, home health facilities, and community speech, language, and hearing centers. If there is a school for the deaf near you, call the staff audiologist for suggestions. In some cases you will not be accepted for testing without a recommendation from your physician. A written recommendation will be helpful if you file for Medicare or any other health insurance program reimbursement.

Audiological Testing   On your first visit the audiologist may engage you in conversation to give you an opportunity to express your concerns about your hearing. When you are asked to describe the difficulty you have been having, you may report that

- the sounds you hear never seem loud enough
- the sound is loud enough, but you don't understand some of the words
- people talk too fast, or they mumble
- you can't stand the background noises
- your family keeps asking you to turn down the television

These initial complaints and others usually surface when people have a mild loss. The audiologist will probably consider not only what you say but also the loudness of your speech and the kind of attention you seem to pay to the face of someone else who is speaking.

A machine called an audiometer can test how well you are hearing sounds produced mechanically. An audiogram, which I will discuss shortly, is used to keep a record of the way you hear a variety of sounds. You may spend a long time—often as much as two hours—on a detailed series of tests to determine where, in your particular case, there has been a breakdown in the complex circuitry of the ear.

The process of hearing starts with a disturbance in the waves of air caused by vibration. Vibrations do not occur in a single pattern, however, like the concentric circles created by a pebble thrown into calm water. The pattern is complicated by the vibration from all the sounds in the environment. It is as if pebbles of differing size were being thrown from a variety of directions, all perceived by the sensitive parts of two small clusters of bones and tissue on opposite sides of the head. Because waves vary in size and in the speed per second at which they travel, we have tone and pitch. Loudness relates to the intensity of the waves as they are lengthened. Pitch (frequency) is the number of vibrations of the waves per second. For example, sound waves caused by a musical instrument that reach the eardrum at approximately 256 waves per second produce a pitch we have learned to recognize as middle C on the piano. When the waves are less frequent—perhaps 128 waves per second—they strike the eardrum below middle C. We hear a sound above middle C when 512 waves per second reach the eardrum.

A loss in our hearing may occur for dozens of reasons. The four basic ones that are usually mentioned in the information from the audiologist's series of tests are briefly explained here. The average person soon becomes familiar with the terms *conductive* and *sensorineural*. Conductive loss is caused by a mechanical difficulty in the way sound is conveyed through the middle ear. The sound fails to travel efficiently through the ear canal, the eardrum, and the tiny bones of the middle ear and into the cochlea. The impairment may result from a blockage, from malformation, or from damage to the outer or middle ear structures. The blockage may have occurred from frequent colds, allergies, or childhood illness; from buildup of wax; or from inflammation or infection in the ear canal. The problem may be hereditary or associated with birth defects. Waves of vibration travel by both bone and air conduction of sound. In conductive hearing loss, sounds never seem loud enough. When sound is amplified sound reaches the cochlea and stimulates the hair cells just as in a normal ear.

We learn from researchers in music history that Beethoven made a personal discovery of bone conduction when he was desperately trying to use his vanishing hearing. He found he could hear by placing one end of a block of wood between his teeth and the other on the piano. How sad it is that his own innocent discovery did not prompt more significant scientific research into "bone hearing." Scientists did not immediately learn how to use the phenomenon to create some of the hearing instruments common today. One contemporary writer with a hearing loss reports that he hears speech well when an oscillator is placed against the bone in the upper right part of his back. (Rosenthal 1975:25). Most people, though, wear bone conduction aids behind their ears.

If your audiologist diagnoses the cause of your loss as conductive, you may consider yourself relatively fortunate. This type of impairment is often treated medically and surgically with good results. Sometimes even total hearing is restored. If for some reason surgery is ruled out, a hearing aid is still a possibility. A mechanical aid is more satisfactory as a means of improving conductive hearing than it would be in other situations because by amplifying the sounds it treats the main cause of distress. Incoming sounds are not distorted with a conductive hearing loss. There is greater tolerance in this type of impairment for loud sounds or background noises, a pervasive source of distress for the elderly, whose impairment almost always reflects sensorineural disturbance.

Sensorineural impairments are commonly known as nerve deafness. In the elderly, nerve deafness is called presbycusis; a sensorineural loss occurs in most people to some degree as they age. The loss is caused by a defect in the inner ear or the auditory nerve. Hair cells embedded in the fluid of the cochlea, connected to some 20,000 to 30,000 nerve fibers, unite through neurons to form the VIIIth nerve (the auditory nerve), which transmits impulses to the brain. The hair cells in the cochlea begin to wear out by age twenty and continue to do so throughout life even though those that remain are collectively strong enough to support four tons of weight per square inch. How the mechanism functions to produce hearing has been in dispute for centuries, and a variety of theories have been explored. The loss involved in presbycusis is usually, although not always, in the high-frequency (high-pitched) sounds. Vowel sounds are better heard and understood than consonant sounds, which may not reach the brain, so that words are often unintelligible.

When hair cells die, there is no replacement. The deterioration may occur faster with some people than with others and accelerates after age sixty. Damage due to the destruction of the cells and the exact point at which such destruction takes place are not easy to determine. There is interference with the vibration of sound waves that determine the intensity as well as the pitch. The impairment becomes noticeable at about age forty, more often in men than in women, usually occurs in both ears, and may be accompanied by tinnitus, noises in the head and some degree of vertigo (dizziness). It is more distressing when there is also the complication of a slight conductive loss.

Aging is not the only cause of presbycusis. Some loss may be conditioned by one's genes or by an inner ear system which is weaker at birth and is susceptible to later deterioration starting in early childhood or at any time thereafter. For example, a child may not experience hearing loss during the first ten or twelve years, but if chronic sinusitis develops, the inner ear may be less capable of withstanding the onslaught and damage that precipitates early loss of hearing.

A long list of diseases may contribute to sensorineural impairment. The New York League for the Hard of Hearing in a brochure prepared by Judith S. May, clinical supervisor in audiology, states that sensorineural loss may be an early symptom of a number of ailments and advises that "good general health care may also result in good hearing health care." The health problems listed as symptomatic are "kidney disease, thyroid problems, arteriosclerosis, diabetes, syphilis and meningitis. Hypertension, heart disease and other vascular problems may affect the blood supply to the hearing mechanism and contribute to damage to the inner ear." Other problems that may entail sensorineural loss include measles, mumps, scarlet fever, diphtheria, whooping cough, influenza, and unidentified virus infection. (These maladies may also be implicated in conductive loss.) Contributing causes which one can hardly avoid in the normal course of living are: prescription drugs, aspirin (taken in large doses and continued for long periods), coffee, tea, and alcohol. Birth defects may also be a cause.

Almost always a major contributing cause is noise exposure. Exposure to intense noises can permanently damage the hair cells. If the noise is extremely intense, like the blast of an explosion, it can actually obliterate sensitivity to sound altogether. Considering the modern extended life span of the elderly, a lifetime of exposure to the proliferating noisy inventions of our industrial civilization will inevitably cause damage. There is evidence that "in populations protected from the noises and other stresses of modern civilization, the effects on hearing that can be attributed to aging per se may be rather negligible" (Newby and Popelka 1985:88).

Currently there is much research and conjecture regarding the effect of poor nutrition on hearing. Some evidence has been reported of the link during a long life between damage in the ear and excessive fats and sodium and inadequate fiber. Such a connection seems likely, inasmuch as other parts of the body are affected by diet. When we reflect on the fact that some degree of nerve deafness may afflict half of the elderly over sixty, and possibly more of those over seventy-five, it becomes clear that the handicap is more and more widespread as this segment of the population increases.

For many years anyone with nerve deafness was told

that a hearing aid would not help and that no other help was available. Fortunately modern technology has solved many mechanical problems and has refined the structure of assistive hearing instruments so that they now provide considerable help for sensorineural impairment, which accounts for perhaps 90 percent of hearing loss among the elderly. And there is the promise of further progress. Digital hearing aids will eventually improve and will help to solve the problem of background noise. Considerable research activity has been stimulated by the competition of many large companies with substantial means. No one today who has been diagnosed as having nerve deafness needs to leave the doctor's office feeling severely discouraged.

Two other sources of impairment are *mixed type*, which is a combination of conductive and sensorineural loss, and *central type*, in which the auditory centers of the brain are affected by injury, disease, tumor, hereditary weakness, presbycusis, or some unknown cause. The problem may not affect the volume of sound but it does impair comprehension.

Comprehensive testing may disclose some physiological condition in the ear that contributes to hearing loss. If a patient has signed a waiver to permit the audiologist to bypass an otologist's test, and the audiologist does find evidence of physical complication, the patient will be advised that a visit with an otologist is essential. Some elderly patients may report being hard of hearing but resist reporting any other troublesome condition in their ears. Their reluctance may stem from fear that their complaints will be attributed to crankiness.

Every publication about the ear that I have read warns about loss due to excessive noise. According to the literature, sudden bursts of noise become even more distressing than a steady noise above 90 decibels; high-pitched sounds are worse than the lower tones. Work becomes less accurate, and quantity is reduced. Most harmful is the fatigue, a reluctance to tackle any peaks in demand, and a loss in incentive.

The Audiometer and the Audiogram   The audiometer was invented in the late nineteenth century and is still commonly used to determine the quantity and quality of a person's hearing. This basic information is then charted on a graph called an audiogram. Audiograms (see figure 2) are kept on file so that any changes in hearing ability can be tracked.

The degree of loudness required for hearing is indicated on the audiogram by the number of decibels (figure 2). Normal hearing of the softest audible sound is marked as −0 decibels to 0 decibels. This is reported as the threshold of hearing in someone who has experienced no loss. Many

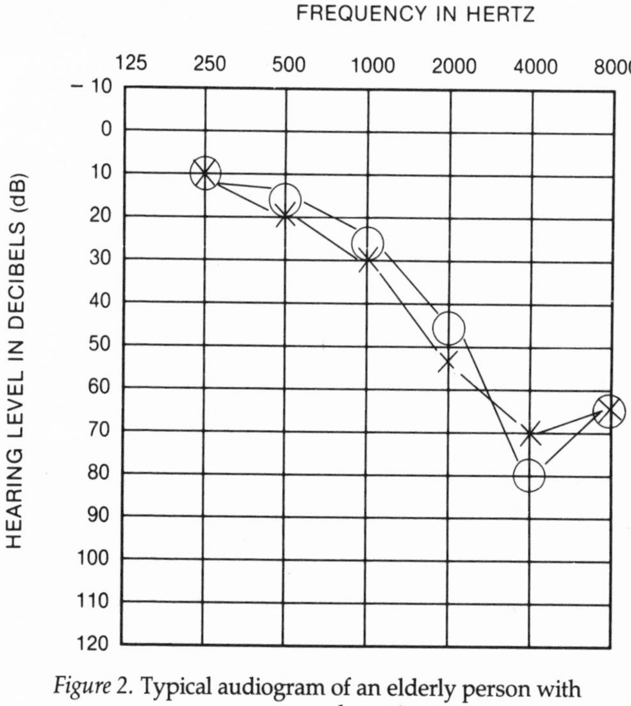

Figure 2. Typical audiogram of an elderly person with sensory presbycusis.

people who are still considered normal in their hearing may not hear a sound until it is raised to 10 or 20 decibels. Those who need amplification greater than 25 decibels are said to be hearing impaired. Those with a threshold of 30 decibels to 45 decibels are said to have a *mild* hearing loss. A *moderate* hearing loss is marked on the audiogram as 45 decibels to 60 decibels; *severe* loss is 60–75 decibels, and a *profound* loss is 75 decibels or more. (There is some variation in the precise figures that audiologists use in making a diagnosis.) Incidentally, rock music is often amplified to 120 decibels and has become a cause of hearing impairment even among teenagers.

Measurements in terms of decibels must also take into account the frequency of sound waves measured in terms of the cycles of vibration per second, or hertz. As the waves of vibration increase—so that there are more cycles of vibration per second—the pitch, or tone, rises. A shrill sound, like the whistle of a kettle, has a high frequency. A low frequency sound has fewer cycles of vibration per second. The human ear will not hear an extremely low hum (low frequency) unless the hum is amplified, that is, unless the decibels of sound are increased. A person with a hearing loss in the high tones, will not hear a high tone sound unless it is amplified.

In the case of speech sounds, there is difficulty in hearing and comprehending consonants like *th*, *f*, *s*, and *t*, because the sound of most consonants is less intense. Vowel sounds are far more easily distinguished. The word "broom," with its strong double vowel sound, may be heard clearly, but pairs such as "sheath" and "seize" will often be interpreted as the same word.

Cycles of sound appear on an audiogram as "frequencies" in a range from about 200 to 8000 hertz. (See figure 2.) Although sounds increase and can be heard by the normal human ear to 20,000 hertz, most normal hearing occurs in the range that the audiogram covers. (Dogs and other animals hear beyond that range, as you may have noticed.) Almost all elderly people with a sensorineural loss have difficulty with the high-frequency sounds. They may not hear the ring of the telephone or the doorbell unless the sound is considerably amplified. They may hear men's low-pitched voices more clearly than the higher-toned voices of women and children. Only a small proportion of people with this kind of loss (presbycusis) do better with the high-pitched sounds and struggle to hear the lower ones. (I am one of these.)

The audiologist tests your hearing loss at 250, 500, 1000, 2000, 4000, and 8000 hertz, beginning with a very loud sound and ending with the softest sound you can hear, which is the "threshold" at which you hear the sound at that particular pitch. A mark is placed on the audiogram showing your threshold of hearing in decibels at each frequency. The audiologist tests each ear separately and marks the results with an O for your right ear and an X for your left ear (see figure 2).

Someone with a loss of 20 decibels (the figure is the average of all the marks on the audiogram) can hear conversation clearly from a distance of as much as fifteen feet, which may be across a room of average size. With a 30 decibel loss a person can still hear from a distance of ten feet; a 40 decibel loss would require the listener to stand six feet from the speaker and a 50 decibel loss would bring the listener to three and one-half feet. Thus you can see that normal conversation may be quite audible despite a considerable loss, especially if the sound is amplified by the use of a hearing aid. My discussion presumes that the speaker is not an inordinately fast talker and does not speak with the lips almost closed or have other habits that require the listeners to increase their attentiveness.

Another condition of hearing loss identified by an audiologist through speech audiometry testing is *discrimination*. This term denotes our ability to understand the words in the sounds we hear. Sound is not absent; it is out of kilter. Human ears hear more than 350,000 separate sounds. The normal ear accomplishes a herculean feat of interpretation. An understanding of the spoken word depends on the adequacy of the higher hearing centers of the brain. Loss in them is sometimes called word deafness but is more commonly termed nerve deafness. Many factors relating to type of impairment affect how well we understand the speech we are hearing. Testing for discrimination involves the use of word lists to record the percentage of words that are correctly identified. The victim of nerve deafness may feel deeply frustrated because, depending on the degree of impairment, total communication breaks down, no matter how loud the sound is that reaches the ears. People afflicted with nerve deafness will therefore often plead "please don't shout"; by talking more loudly the well-intentioned speaker adds to the difficulty of understanding. The problem of discrimination makes it harder to derive maximum benefit from a hearing aid. Partly for this reason many people, after investing time and money in a hearing aid, retreat from the conflict of adjustment and stash their instrument in a bureau drawer along with other precious jewels.

Normal tolerance and high discrimination scores would ordinarily represent conductive impairment, but some patients with sensorineural impairment have speech audiometric scores indistinguishable from those of conductively impaired patients. It is therefore risky to attempt a complete diagnosis from speech audiometric tests alone (Newby and Popelka 1985:180–81).

The Hearing Instrument Dealer/Specialist

Hearing aid sales offices have proliferated and are now present in every sizable community. They usually advertise free hearing tests and offer a long list of services that may tempt you to bypass an appointment with an otologist and an audiologist. The tests are administered by the dealers, who often receive their training from the hearing aid companies whose products they sell. Audiologists who do not sell aids refer their patients to a dealer, with whom they work cooperatively to help each patient learn to use the aid. Visit an audiologist rather than accepting a dealer's offer to provide audiometric testing, especially if the dealer sells only one company's product.

The National Hearing Aid Society is an association for certified hearing instrument specialists. This group provides its members with opportunities to increase their level of proficiency and competency by completing a stringent certification process, continuing education requirements, and educational seminars. The society also advocates the establishment of a national board of certification in hearing instrument sciences. (See appendix 4 for the address and telephone number.) An audiologist who has on hand a variety of hearing aids that you can try in order to make a selection will of course prefer to sell you an aid. If you have been tested in a professional center or by an individual audiologist, and neither one sells hearing aids, you will usually be given the name of a dealer, or several, leaving you free to make your own selection. The center or audiologist will want to check the performance of the aid during the trial period.

An aid purchased from a dealer can mean that the dealer has an important responsibility in follow-up, more so if he or she has some form of certified training. For many weeks, in some cases months, you will be struggling to adjust to a whole new way of life with an ingenious and somewhat mysterious apparatus. Trained dealers can make adjustments when you report some difficulty. They are often less pressured and show patience and concern in serving you.

You can purchase new batteries from a dealer and feel assured that they will be fresh and of good quality.

There is a great temptation to succumb to the enthusiastic salesmanship of some dealers. I know that some people have had satisfactory experience with them and are especially grateful when competition means that lower prices are charged for the same standard model. Bear in mind, however, that the audiologist is professionally trained to provide a more comprehensive program of treatment beyond the initial evaluation and selection of hearing aids.

It is clear from the discussion above that many factors must be considered in assessing the nature of an impairment and in determining the kind of help that mechanical devices may provide. Many factors other than the degree of loss indicated on an audiogram affect a person's ability to hear. They include the personality of the hearer; care in listening; effort and persistence; skill in speechreading and in interpreting gestures, facial expressions, dialects, and accents; the extent to which ability to concentrate can overcome the distraction of peripheral sounds; relative interest in the subject; physical condition (illness or debility may drain energy); and in every case the acoustics in the environment. In short, two people whose audiograms appear similar may vary considerably in their success at managing their handicap.

The audiologist determines the degree of hearing loss by studying the audiogram. While one audiologist may call a 40 decibel loss mild, however, another may call it mild to moderate. Moreover, human beings don't function with the precision of machines. Behavior varies from day to day, even hourly. You may be more alert during one examination, or more tired, or low in mood, or worried and tense about your condition. I find that my hearing varies with the weather, perhaps because of air pressure. On clear, bright, sunny days I feel more alert and seem to be hearing better. In foggy or cloudy weather, I have a sense of thickness in the air that seems to impede my hearing. Since I am excessively sensitive to cold temperature, I don't relax in a room where the thermometer registers below 70 degrees. The results of a test in this case might indicate a greater loss than if I had been tested in a 75 degree room, in which I feel pleasantly relaxed. Such subjective reactions may well affect the audiometric reading. An audiogram, therefore, while certainly a useful indicator of how well you can hear, should not be the only device used to diagnose your condition.

Competent audiologists are trained to use their experience to consider all these related factors, treating the total person rather than focusing narrowly on the mechanical function of hearing during a test. It is therefore advisable to continue to visit the same audiologist for the annual tests and consultation, just as one sees the same medical doctor at regular intervals. An otologist, if one is used, should also remain the same over a period of years.

THREE

My First Full Examination

The nickname *Traümerin* stayed with me throughout my childhood, and other evidence of my tendency to daydream entered the catalog of stories recounted during family reunions. I recall, for instance, the incident that led to the comment "Charlotte's catching flies again." One day when Mama called us in for lunch, she had prepared a rare treat of assorted cold cuts purchased at a German delicatessen. This was a culinary treat in our austere household, where stewed prunes were considered fit for dessert. One of my older sisters surveyed the table and asked, "Mama, could we have pickles too?" She meant the dripping and pungent half-sour pickles that were taken from a barrel of brine in the store. We used to buy them for a penny.

Mama had a ready excuse. "Someone would have to go out to get them." I was marching around the big oak kitchen table, swinging a fly swatter, adrift in my own thoughts, when I heard my sister say, "Charlotte will go." Like the dutiful middle child that I was, I left on my errand without protest, not even stopping to return the fly swatter to its hook on the kitchen closet door. Just outside the deli was a huge beef truck, its rear doors damp and sticky, riddled with the biggest flies I had ever seen. They were sluggish, as if sated. It would be wicked fun to lift my murderous fly swatter against such somnolent insects, giants of their species, sparkling in the brilliant summer sun. I advanced upon them as in a dream, enchanted by the listless behavior of a horde of normally nimble creatures. Much time passed before I finally woke up and remembered my errand. I ran home in addled confusion, still clutching the nickel in my warm fist.

The kitchen shone in pristine cleanliness, the fancy embroidered tablecloth having been replaced with the one we ordinarily used for meals. Nothing remained of the recent repast. Apparently lunch had been fully consumed, but still Mama asked, "Where are the pickles?"

I stared at the coin in my hand and hastily fabricated a reply to conceal my shame. "They cost ten cents. The storekeeper said to go home and get another nickel." Noting the fly swatter still drooping from my hand, one of my sisters howled, "Träumerin! You were out there for a whole hour catching flies!" Thereafter, whenever I was caught dreaming by a family member, I would get a nudge and the reminder, "Träumerin! Stop catching flies!" Later my lapses into a private world became a romantic manifestation of my poetry-writing adolescence and seemed quite normal. My family left off nudging me back into reality, but to this day I tend to slip into dreamy reverie from time to time.

Well into adulthood, as my hearing began to deteriorate, I reverted often to fantasies. Efforts to hear other people so that I could participate in conversations created exhausting stress during extended social functions. I withdrew, as I had in my childhood, but reverie now became a form of release when I was tired and sought relaxation and renewal.

A few years ago, after I had had tests and consultations with a number of different audiologists, one of them said, "Yours is the kind of hearing loss that is due, not only to the presbycusis of aging, but also to a defect you must have had way back in early childhood." If this particular diagnosis was correct, then it would explain two much later occasions when my behavior was criticized.

On my first office job when I was just out of college and naive and tense, I kept making foolish mistakes, especially in handling telephone messages. A sympathetic supervisor once chided me gently with the remark, "The trouble with you, Charlotte, is that you don't seem to listen." The words scared me because I felt that she was right.

The second incident tucked away among my memories concerns a sewing lesson I was being given by a friend. I kept ignoring her instructions, messing up the seams of a pair of white linen slacks. Finally she took the fabric from me and began carefully to pull out the errant threads. Shaking her head, she remarked,

"The trouble with you, Charlotte, is that you have no patience. I keep trying to tell you something, and you don't pay any attention to what I'm saying."

It may be, of course, that neither of these incidents bears any relation to my later difficulties. When I related them to another audiologist he shrugged his shoulders and said, "We just don't know. There's no way of telling." But such recollections stay with me. In today's enlightened times, when I read about the hearing tests administered by school nurses, I hail the advance and voice my support.

A number of national organizations are now working to erase the stigma of hearing impairment and to lure the afflicted back from their private worlds. They encourage us to be candid and self-respecting. They explore the role of the family, promote self-help and support groups, and provide information about the technological advances, including new forms of assistive listening devices and training in speechreading and in listening. They study the extensive research that offers new hope for those with afflicted hearing. Later I will describe my discovery of Self Help for Hard of Hearing People (SHHH), which was the breakthrough that changed the whole direction of my life.

For a long time, as all the sounds of my world grew softer and subdued, I was unconsciously using my compensatory skills. I became watchful, vigilantly attentive. Some people were flattered by my concentration on what they were saying, although I sometimes seemed to be staring. (They stared back!) Occasionally I noticed that someone would become uncomfortable and would turn away slightly as we conversed. I worked at managing my need to concentrate on the face of the speaker without causing discomfort or even shyness. More and more often I raised my voice louder than necessary and was quickly hushed by friends. On some occasions when this happened I felt ashamed and remained quiet for some time before resuming participation in the conversation. Because I could not gauge how loud my own voice was, I often raised it in order to hear it at the level of loudness that seemed normal to me. Unfortunately, this level was much louder than that required by people with normal hearing.

Much of the process of loss that I have described had already occurred before I was brave enough to concede that I had a hearing problem. In time I realized that I could not continue to suppress the knowledge—from myself or from others—that many more sounds "out there" were lost to my awareness. The need for acceptance had overcome my need for denial and resistance.

The decision I had made after six years to be open and honest about my hearing impairment was implemented only in stages, beginning with my small family. I also managed to acknowledge my problem in impersonal encounters with strangers, store clerks, mailmen, and solicitors—people I was not likely to see frequently. But with friends and other relatives I continued to stumble along a rutted road of pretense. I was convinced that they already knew. I shrank from confronting a problem that had been veiled by mutual agreement. To talk about it would condemn me as someone who was "handicapped." Although communication at home continued within the shelter of a family truce, the freedom of normal rapport sustained during these difficult years was constantly threatened. I didn't want to be "different." I didn't want people to "make allowances," to have to change their words, to scrutinize my face to see whether I had heard, to say things twice to avoid misinterpretation. Already one friend had begun to interrupt her conversation to ask, "Did you hear me?" Such maneuvers would be helpful, but I was afraid to pay the price. I knew I would have to leap over the hurdle someday.

I luxuriated in the balm of affection and tenderness of my husband and my daughter, for now we were as one, open to the requirements of my loss. We had become a team accepting its demands. It was helpful to be able to allude to the trouble I was having in the privacy of our home, to ask for help, to be spoken to in a voice carefully modulated in pace and intensity, to leave it to the one who was around when the phone rang to deal with a request or message that could be handled without my intervention. These were no small concessions, and I was sustained for a while longer. I was becoming more knowledgeable about the ear's eccentricities. Lou and Susan waited patiently for some time while I promised to secure reliable audiometric testing as soon as I had found the best source.

One day when we were invited to an evening party with friends I made some excuse not to arrive early. After three hours I poked my husband's arm and pointed to my wristwatch, a signal that I wanted to leave. I could tell he was embarrassed at having to make the first move to break up a congenial gathering so soon. Deftly he succeeded in inventing a reason that would forestall the pleading of our surprised hostess.

As soon as we were outside I felt revived by the cool night breeze and refreshed by the quiet of a dark suburban street. A silver moon silhouetted leaves against the night sky. I found the world beautiful, polished clear of human sound and confusion.

"Why did you want to leave so early?"

"I was tired. There was so much noise, I missed things they were saying, and I was afraid to participate. What if I should say something that would seem stupid and they'd all laugh?"

"But you were getting along fine."

"That's just it. I didn't want to spoil it." And I added with a laugh, "You know—quit while I was still ahead."

We lapsed into an uneasy quiet on our walk back home. My heels clicked lightly against the pavement. I heard the bark of a dog once, but no other sounds broke the restful silence. Did he guess how much I regretted having spoiled a pleasant evening for him, how baffled I was, and how I now wished I hadn't wanted to leave early? He betrayed no disappointment; when I gallantly resolved to be open about my loss he had become my ally, but when I set limits on my openness, I made him another victim of my irresolution.

I had done the same thing to my daughter, Susan. One day we asked her to join us for a party at a dinner theater. The play that we were to see was a short comedy performed on a platform before the diners. Anticipating my needs, Susan asked the hostess beforehand, without my knowledge, to seat us close to the performers. When several of the actors mounted the improvised stage close by, carrying their musical instruments, I knew I was in for trouble. I sat through the performance without understanding anything—neither the words of the actors nor the conversation at the table. I looked longingly at several empty seats in the rear but resisted as overly conspicuous the impulse to move back to escape the noise. Susan had taken pleasure in planning for me to enjoy the play. Not wanting to disappoint her I refrained from admitting that I was totally ignorant of what was going on and tried to look intelligent as she conversed with her father.

Other incidents acted to push me toward my stated goal. In the entertainment section of the Sunday *Times*, my husband found an announcement of subscription programs for a series of plays that "we should be getting tickets for." I failed to respond to the suggestion because it was becoming more difficult for me to grasp what was happening on the stage. Going to the theater with friends was socially trying, especially as it usually included much animated discussion during intermission and afterward. I would have to be careful about my own contributions to such conversations, since I would not fully have understood the play. What often made it worse was when the actors spoke in dialect or used words in a foreign language or affected a carefree casual style. My seat seemed to be miles away. Moreover, during a performance the audience seemed to be full of coughers and of people tearing at crisp cellophane candy wrappers, whispering to neighbors, rustling programs, or using fans. My husband, who truly loves the theater, was disappointed when I declined invitations to accompany our friends. It was embarrassing to keep refusing them, but we found some reasons to use: a conflict in dates, a recent illness, visits of families with children due sometime soon. Paradoxically, however, when they stopped asking us I missed their overtures even while I was relieved at not having to decline.

To keep these cherished friendships alive, we often arranged dinners at a restaurant. There I fussed about the location of our table, a particular annoyance to my amiable husband, who was always contented no matter where we sat. When we were a party of eight, I refused the first table offered, which was long and narrow, and asked for the only round table I could see, which, as it turned out, had another party's "reserved" sign on it. At various other times I objected to a table in the middle of a large room where we would be surrounded by other diners, especially if their voices had risen over a round of drinks. I insisted on good lighting so that I could gather speech clues from faces. I shook my head vigorously when we were ushered to a table near the entrance or in any other place with heavy traffic, for example near the bar or the spot where a busboy stood behind a counter, piling dishes and clinking silver. I felt uneasy, even impatient with the others in our party because they had left it to me to contend with the hostess, whose smile was fading fast.

When we finally sat down, I did not dare call attention to the flickering candle in the center of the table or the vase of flowers that cut into my view of everyone in our party. By this time I was dreadfully ashamed of my behavior. We placed our orders. Once my husband stopped me from interrupting when I failed to observe that someone else was still talking to the waiter. Soon new diners were arriving noisily. Almost nothing intelligible penetrated my brain except an occasional phrase that teased me until I was limp from the effort to stay in touch. Swirls of movement behind me, the clamor of rattling dishes, obtrusive "background" music jangling in my ears, the exhaust fan or air conditioner—all seemed to be burying me. In the midst of so much activity I was alone, but I ached to be part of it. Worst of all, there were sudden bursts of laughter. I had two choices in this setting: I could remain utterly still and try to look as though I understood, or I could launch into speech that would hold others captive as they listened. But the latter choice was hazardous as I risked alluding to something that had already been discussed. My voice was often too loud, and at such times Lou warned me with a gesture to lower it.

To offset the strain of such occasions, I arranged small gatherings for coffee and dessert at our home. The closeness at these times enabled me to match up others' gestures and facial expressions with the verbal sounds I could hear quite clearly. Besides, now that my faithful ally at my side knew of my loss, I felt protected. Nevertheless I was content when the first of my guests made some sign that they wanted to leave early. I wonder now whether they noticed that I produced coats and handbags with alacrity as others rose to follow them. I enjoyed the evenings and I could tell that my guests did too, but when quiet settled in our home after the flurry of farewells I felt relief. I had committed no blunders; we parted warmly with genuine embraces. I felt keenly that our lives had been blessed with the gift of lasting friendships.

One day I came upon an arresting passage in Jane Howard's biography of Margaret Mead. In her late seventies the famous anthropologist "had suffered one of the most crippling of infirmities; she could no longer hear all that people around her were saying. . . . After lectures she no longer took questions from the floor. All her life she had made the best of physical ailments. . . . But (partial) deafness was another matter" (Howard 1984:481–82). These words alerted me to a number of other statements in Howard's intensely researched story of Margaret Mead. In her early twenties, for example, breathless with the excitement of her new life as a student of anthropology, she wrote home from Samoa of "a curious buzzing noise inside one's head, mostly from the strain of listening."

This sentence leaped off the page at me. I connected her remarks with what I had only recently learned about buzzing noises inside the head. Her problem may have been an omen of tinnitus, the bane of half the elderly with presbycusis. Indeed, when she was in her seventies, her niece remarked that she had become "very cranky" and that "hearing trouble was making her very nervous" (Howard 1984:415). "Did she sense that something much more ominous was going on inside her?" asks Jane Howard.

I wondered, too, when I read in Howard's biography, "Her lifelong tendency to come straight to the point, a blunt and refreshing impatience, turned now to plain, and sometimes astonishing, rudeness." This tendency was intensified by the distress and apprehension she endured from the strain of a devastating impairment, the more so because obviously she had kept the news of her affliction from the public and even from her colleagues. Ironically, it was helpful to me to learn that I was not unique in my attitude toward my problem.

I still enjoyed attending concerts where social interaction seemed to be muted. People who love classical music are less talkative in a concert hall than people are at the theater. If I chose to keep quiet during intermissions, or even afterward, I felt that social withdrawal in this environment was no imposition on my companions. As soon as I had settled into my seat, I shed the bonds of the day's tight control. Listening to music I experienced unalloyed rapture, because although I missed some sounds, I could hear and respond to the rhythmical vibrations, which penetrated the dead cells in my inner ear. Whatever I could not hear well was far less than all that I did hear. The music came as a nourishing banquet to my starving senses. I made the discovery that people who attended these concerts listen with absorption rarely broken by coughs and the crackling of paper. Moreover, as my acuity diminished, I sharpened my listening skills, a most welcome form of compensation. I could hear and enjoy the distinctive sounds of a flute or oboe solo, the clarinet, and the English horn. The tuba and the bass fiddle seemed now more richly a part of the symphonic composite, and the haunting notes of the cello hung fresh and poignant in the air.

At home we moved our hi-fi into the living room, had it cleaned and reconditioned, and used the finest needles. Our favorite records and tapes were scattered about. I learned to conquer my housekeeping compulsion to fight the clutter.

During the ensuing months, while I was still uneasily preparing to take the decisive step and confront an audiologist, I became more troubled by the many small irritations of each day. When I sat beside my husband in the car, still a treasured luxury at that time, I noticed the slightest unusual sound in its performance. "Something's whistling," I might report, or "Don't you hear that click?" He slowed the car and strained to hear. "Nothing's wrong. Stop fussing." But the next day it was his turn. "I hear a little thump when I speed up the motor to sixty. Listen, and tell me if you hear it." I couldn't, which puzzled him. Not until after my evaluation by an audiologist did I learn that my hearing was close to normal for the high-pitched sounds but defective in the low-pitched area, an unusual type of impairment for someone with presbycusis, while my husband, conversely, had a very slight hearing loss that is considered much more common among people over seventy for the same high-pitched sounds. The disparity produced some animated conversation, since we were unable to convince each other that our precious car was misbehaving.

I drew scant comfort from the fact that people with normal hearing can make similar mistakes. When I informed someone that I had lived in Teaneck for thirty years, he commented, "Really? I had no idea you came from so far west as Phoenix." He had not heard the high-pitched consonant sound of the *t* and had not observed the movement of my lips, which would have been different for pronouncing an *f* as in "Phoenix." Had he been a speechreader, like most hard-of-hearing people, he might not have misunderstood me. He heard "eenix" and "eeneck," which sounded identical to his ears. If I had made the same mistake I would have felt apologetic. He did not, and I envied him.

It would have helped me to know that my vacillation about freely acknowledging my problem was common to everyone in this predicament. Unlike visual handicaps, a hearing impairment appears to be a personality deviation and is so regarded by strangers. I have often thought about the first time I met Bill, who became one of our dearest friends. I used to see this slim, six-foot-two-inch blonde Adonis flash by as I took my morning walk near our Florida home. He would stop by the pool for a short swim, towel his taut, narrow-hipped form efficiently, then promptly disappear. Once I tried to hold him with a smile and acknowledgment, but I received scant response before he resumed his solitary course with his characteristic graceful stride.

"Who's that guy?" I asked my husband. "I'd like to talk to him. He doesn't *look* unfriendly but he seems sort of anxious to get away."

"I know. I've noticed that too. Don't keep annoying him; he's strange."

But I persisted. One day I came upon him in the spa, diligently pulling at the oars on the rowing machine. He greeted me warmly and removed the instrument covering his ears. "I've been listening to my favorite musical program—comes on at this time every morning."

That was a felicitous beginning. Soon we were conversing about a subject of mutual interest. The spa was a quiet place at that hour, with excellent acoustics and insulated against outside noises. Bill explained that his hearing was impaired, but in this environment it presented no problem. (Later I learned that he was a superb speech- and lipreader. I will have more to say about people like Bill. After my hearing had deteriorated further, I met many other speechreaders who came to the workshops that I introduced for the benefit of the hard of hearing.)

The impression that my husband and I both had initially had that there was "something strange" about Bill became an unpleasant memory. Later I too grew wary of seeming to appear "strange." I consoled myself with the hope that, if I "went public," as I had resolved to do, I would be spared such humiliation. Years passed before I could take the first step of sharing my predicament with my immediate family and with strangers. I wish I had known that my behavior was typical. Instead of admitting "I don't hear very well," people who are hard of hearing genuinely believe it when they say "You're mumbling" or "Your voice is too low." I was determined to avoid such self-delusion; I needed to feel socially acceptable, and denying my problem had only prevented it. Privately I could not get rid of the harsh judgment that I was somehow at fault for not having heard the speaker. ("Sorry . . . I missed what you just said.") Sorry, sorry, sorry. Backing against a wall of self-condemnation was no way to build self-esteem! Worse yet was a gnawing suspicion that everyone could see through my attempts to dissemble. ("Your best friends won't tell you.")

When President Reagan's hearing had to be fortified with a hearing aid, and the news media seized on the information, I welcomed the publicity, expecting it to bring greater public understanding of the invisible handicap. With my sharpened skill in noting who was hard of hearing, however, I saw that nothing had changed for those who kept their disability a secret. The additional information that Reagan was wearing two hearing aids and not just one underscored the idea that he could acknowledge his impairment without fear of any consequences. I mused on the ironic fact that he could boldly reveal his hearing loss, while millions of others still hid theirs for fear of how they might be treated.

Not until both Lou and Susan assumed an aggressive stance was I finally to promise them that I would follow through. No sooner had I done so than they embarked on a campaign of constant prodding:

"*When* are you going to get your hearing taken care of?"

"If you cannot hear me, why don't you get a hearing aid?"

"Don't blame me if you got our date wrong."

"It's not fair to lean on other people to keep straightening out your mistakes."

Finally Susan gave me the dreaded brush-off: "You'd better let me talk to Dad, Mom."

I had been enjoying the freedom at home after leaving the closet, and at last I stepped out further.

First I allowed the news to filter out to other members of our large family. There was a surge of phone calls daily. I learned that no one was surprised to learn of my hearing loss. My relatives had known about it all along! They poured out suggestions, gossip about other people with similar afflictions, and so forth. I discovered I actually enjoyed their involvement. Their expressions of concern were so nurturing and enthusiastic. Why had I clung for so many years to secrecy and denial?

(Years later, when I had become dedicated to helping hearing-impaired people, I was able to console many of them who felt ashamed of their ambivalence. I understood that for them to quit stalling would mean to accept the dreaded diagnosis as final and to accept the reality that nothing could bring about a refurbishing of an ear's worn-out parts, that to be hard of hearing was forever.)

Two of my sisters said they knew "someone" who had had some contact with the New York League for the Hard of Hearing. The very name of the organization had a ring of authority and sincerity that attracted me. The location was easy to reach from my home in Teaneck, New Jersey. In a telephone call, I was informed that the league sponsored a program of professional hearing evaluation, consultation, and guidance for corrective solutions but was not in the business of selling hearing aids. If its evaluation indicated that I would benefit from an aid, I could try several that the league kept on hand from different manufacturers. I could make my own decision as to which worked best for me. I could then purchase a similar aid from any dealer on the league's approved list, or from any I chose to patronize elsewhere, and the league would administer another brief test with it to corroborate that my selection had been sound.

Information came pouring through the wires—exactly the kind of details I needed. What's more, the speaker had evidently had training in using the telephone effectively with hard-of-hearing callers. How sweet it was to be able to hear her so easily! I eagerly arranged for an appointment.

As soon as I saw the woman who was to administer the basic interview and evaluation, I had the sensation that the long hard years of denial and deception had come to an end. The room was neat, and the acoustics sustained only the level of sound one might encounter in a quiet home. The clear-eyed young woman who was to devote the next two hours to my welfare greeted me crisply and smiled as she introduced herself. "I'm Ashley Baker," she said, taking my hand. I even liked the romantic sound of her name. Such positive first impressions eroded the tightness I had been feeling. Ashley Baker's deft but gentle manner seemed right for me.

"Has your hearing been giving you much of a problem lately?"

"Now it does. You bet! Especially at home," I said. "It's my husband who is really having the problem there. And when my daughter visits, she minds a lot." I smiled, to cover up the hurt of telling.

She nodded. "I'm not surprised. Often it's the one you live with who wants the help."

She reached for some equipment and described the kind of tests she was about to administer. The standard instruments which she was about to use have some limitations, as I later learned. The audiometer, which is used to acquire the scientific information recorded on an audiogram, is a useful device but not an infallible one; however, if properly calibrated, it yields reliable information. The readings also reflect the vicissitudes of human responses. I had an opportunity to see how testing results varied some time later in different situations. I was tested twice in one week by different audiologists on different equipment with different results. Perhaps my energy was not as high during the second test. Perhaps I was affected by the humidity in the air, which had changed, or I was feeling more relaxed the second time. Like variations in blood pressure, audiometric changes cannot be avoided. The best an audiologist can do is to repeat parts of the test for verification. A competent, sensitive practitioner knows when to check the results that are coming through and to minimize the inconsistencies.

Ashley Baker prepared me carefully for what she was about to do. "I'm going to fit earphones over each ear. I'll be testing one ear at a time. First I'll find the softest sound you are able to hear. Signal to me by raising your hand when I've struck a sound which you have just begun to hear. I'll keep making the sound louder gradually. Raise your hand as you hear each sound. After a certain point, I'll go back and lower it gradually until you indicate by not raising your hand that you can no longer hear it. I'll repeat this several times, until I'm sure how much sound I need to apply in order for you to hear. I'll make a record on your audiogram of this point. We'll go through the same process with the other ear. I'll then have some record of whether you hear sounds better with one ear than with the other." This was essentially the basic approach during the first series of tests. The audiogram then showed the threshold level of my ability to hear sounds, both for "intensity" (loudness) and "frequency" (tone or pitch).

The next series of tests involved speech audiometry. Ashley Baker moved into an adjoining room where we could observe each other through a closed window. Wiring enabled her to hear and record my voice. Her own voice reached me at a variety of sound levels that were controlled through her use of a microphone attached to an audiometer. The first exercise was to test my ability to repeat words correctly from a standard word list as her voice became softer and softer. She instructed me to repeat each two-syllable word after hearing it through her microphone. The exercise seemed childish at first, and I enjoyed being able to breeze through it.

But the next exercise used a list of words that challenged my skill, especially as I had no way of knowing whether I had made an error. She spoke with a card covering the lower part of her face. Unable to watch her lips I realized for the first time how much I had become dependent on my eyes to bolster my faltering hearing. It startled me to discover how this change had become a fixture in my style of communication. When I was unable to see half of her face, I had the illusion that her whole person had receded to some dim area several feet further from me. In chapter 2 I explained how higher frequencies are required to hear consonants. I wasn't sure whether I had heard "sat" or "fat" or "hat," since each of these simple words begins and ends with a consonant and requires a higher frequency than such words as "room" or "load," which have strong vowel sounds. This was one of the areas now being tested.

My score on these word lists would reveal how well I could distinguish the words that were spoken to me and whether the words would be processed in my brain and would become intelligible. It related to a frustration I experienced all day long, when I tried to understand what I heard with background noises present. Over and over, Lou would ask, "Can't you hear that? It seems loud enough." At such times I would explain, "I *do* hear it, but I can't figure out what the sounds mean. And please don't shout at me. That only makes it worse." Technically this is described as "discrimination" which I discussed briefly earlier. It is the most plaintive lament of the elderly who are hard of hearing.

Some 16 million to 20 million of us, according to the statistics, are trying to stay connected to our surroundings in spite of a handicap that others are incapable of fully appreciating because, more than "hard of hearing," it means "hard to understand."

There was no physical discomfort or pain involved in taking the tests. For some time I felt composed and interested and thoroughly relaxed. But after a while I tired of the discipline needed to focus on a battery of tests, to take orders and obey instructions. I had begun to struggle with the harder word list, and I felt unreasonably afraid I was making too many errors. I wish I had known then, as I floundered, that the list allowed for a wide margin of error. On a fifty-word list, I could have made ten errors and still have registered a discrimination score equivalent to only a mild hearing loss. For over an hour I had behaved obediently. I wanted to believe that I was responding honestly to the instructions, but sometimes it seemed to me that I had yielded to a temptation to cheat by saying I heard a sound when perhaps I had not. Did my need to come up with a better "report card" influence my reaction? Sitting in the chair, quietly obeying "teacher," had evoked an image of childhood. I wanted desperately to pass the tests with high marks as in my schoolgirl days, to be praised for being right, to be told I didn't have much of a problem. I wanted the whole day's efforts to end with cheery reassurance.

With deft but gentle motions, Ashley Baker removed the paraphernalia around my ears, allowing me a few minutes to enjoy the freedom as she reviewed the records of the examination. When she pulled up a chair and sat down next to me, I watched her face—a smile! Now came the time I had dreamed about for years, when some maternal guardian would satisfy my longing to gain control of the unpredictable performance of one of my senses, someone who was both kind and knowledgeable. I smiled in anticipation.

"The news about your left ear is pretty good," she said. "Your loss is quite mild. Your right ear is giving you more trouble."

(Keep smiling!)

"Your loss there is 40 decibels. That's still a moderate loss, but a hearing aid would help a lot. Do you want to try it?"

"Of course." (That didn't hurt much . . ., did it?)

"The other good news is your discrimination score. It's 85 to 90 percent of normal, so you probably don't have a problem understanding speech."

(Wrong! Not understanding speech is the *worst* thing I've got. . . . Don't tell!)

"A hearing aid will raise the sound level of your hearing. Let's see."

She reached for a magic little box in a drawer. The hearing aid inside consisted of a plain beige pink plastic crescent, with a tube about six inches long from which a smaller bit of curiously shaped plastic dangled (see figure 3). It seemed an innocuous little gadget no more impressive than a baby's toy, but when she inserted the small mold snugly in my ear and did something to it with one finger the room seemed to come alive. I sat there like Alice in Wonderland, now conscious of the wide, wide world of sound. Formerly the room had seemed to me noiseless. Now I could hear a loose sheet on a desk rustling in a current of air. Outside the closed door footsteps passed by. On the other side of the window something mechanical was whirring in the street. I moved and heard my arm brush against the fabric of my skirt, a rough poplin.

"How does my voice sound to you now?" she asked.

I jumped.

"Too loud? Here, I'll turn it down."

Together we played with the volume switch for a few minutes until I was satisfied with the sound level of her

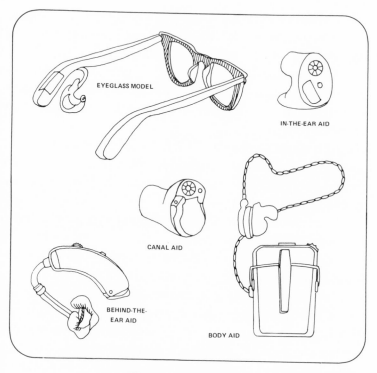

EYEGLASS MODEL

IN-THE-EAR AID

CANAL AID

BEHIND-THE-
EAR AID

BODY AID

Figure 3. Hearing aids.

voice. The rich clarity of her speech with this amplification invaded the stillness. I suddenly remembered when I possessed the ability to hear pure tones and cadences in my surroundings. She moved the switch with her finger back and forth so that I could hear the sound go up or down. When she raised the power, I could feel my heart pounding through the bony structure of my skull. Never had I been so aware of my loss as during these first moments of liberation from it.

"How is it now?"

"Good Lord! It's marvelous! It's wonderful! It's terrific!" I searched for the right words. The sudden sharpness of my voice split the air. I grinned so broadly my face felt taut. I longed to throw my arms around this angel whose ministrations had wrought such a miracle.

"Let's try a few different ones," she said, removing the first aid. I managed to sober down as she fetched several from a drawer. One by one I experimented with their performance. Whatever difference there might have been seemed so insignificant that I wasn't sure I could distinguish any, but I finally chose a particular one, more out of eagerness to get on with the process than from any conviction.

Ms. Baker gave me a copy of my audiogram and furnished a list of dealers to contact, although she said I might be just as successful elsewhere. Perhaps a dealer where I lived would give me a better price than the dealers on her list, who were situated in the heart of the city.

"The important thing to remember," she cautioned, "is that when you do make a purchase you are granted a thirty-day trial period, during which you could return here for me to check your hearing with the instrument you've chosen." If I needed to return the aid, she said, I would be required to pay for the mold that the dealer had had to make, since that was a personal item that would be useless to others.

Often, for my shopping tours, I had gone to the northern New Jersey shopping malls to avoid the steep prices in New York City. The closest New Jersey dispenser of hearing aids was located in a Hackensack mall. Like all such dealers, this one had a substantial supply of testing equipment, but he cordially checked over my report from the New York League and agreed to follow the audiologist's recommendations, providing only the limited service I requested.

He had on hand the same model I had chosen at the New York League as well as a number of others which he suggested I try. He noted that, since the mold on these was not personally prepared, it might not fit perfectly.

"Don't expect the best performance from these trials,"

he said. "You'll get better results once the aid is connected to a mold we make here to fit into your own ear canal."

I was still so enamored by my first experience that I persisted in favoring my first choice. Impatient to possess it, I ignored all previous advice and impulsively decided to end my investigation right then. The dealer lost no time in responding to my choice, promptly proceeding to stuff my ear with some gummy material to form the mold, which was to be attached by a tube to the aid that would rest behind my ear.

"I'll have it for you in two weeks," he promised. It seemed a long time to wait. Already impatient, I paid my deposit, signed a form setting forth the terms of the trial period and the warranty, and left, tingling with excitement.

When I returned two weeks later I reached for the new aid gingerly and tried to follow the dealer's instructions about how to mount it snugly behind my ear and find the comfortable groove for the mold. I was surprised to discover how difficult it was for me. It had seemed so simple when Ashley Baker did it, but now the ear mold kept slipping out.

The dealer smiled patiently. "You're getting nervous," he said. "Look, don't work at it. It goes in easier if you take it easy."

I had to practice much more than I felt should have been necessary, taking it out and inserting it many times before I could tell that I had it fastened securely where it belonged. When I gave him my check and prepared to leave, he took the aid back and replaced it in its little blue velvet box, handed it to me with a sheaf of interesting literature about care of hearing aids, and cautioned me about how to start using it.

"Don't try to wear it out in the street yet. I'd suggest you try it only at home for a few days, where it's quieter."

"Oh, but it's so much trouble getting it on," I demurred. "I'm going to put it on and keep it there just this time."

"Suit yourself," he said with a shrug. I opened the box,

so like a jewel case, and carefully removed the gem. He watched, smiling and nodding, as I arranged it correctly around my ear.

Upstairs, going out of the mall to the busy parking area, I received a shock. The world had become a circus of noises: trucks pounding on the bumpy asphalt, horns honking, passersby shouting, children screeching, music blasting out of nowhere. Quickly I reduced the power with my finger, as I had been instructed, down to almost zero. The silence was a relief, but I kept turning it up again, playing with it greedily like a baby with a new toy.

I spent the next fifteen minutes walking about before boarding a bus to the city subway across the bridge. I kept fiddling with my gadget, locating the degree of sound I thought I might endure on a subway platform. I loved the sudden sense of power I acquired by being able to control sound in my environment.

In the crowded subway car I stood shakily, blanketed in muffled thunder as I hung onto the strap for balance. I had to turn the power of the aid down completely. My right ear began to itch from the unaccustomed contact of the plastic mold. This is a good time, I thought, to prove to myself that I could face up to wearing a hearing aid in public. I shoved the strap of my bag over my shoulder and, with my legs braced against the jolt of the subway train, I removed the mold and earpiece and rubbed my cheek and ear vigorously to relieve the itching. Then I fumbled for several minutes trying to replace the equipment. I sensed that I had aroused the curiosity of the man next to me, who clung, swaying, to his strap. Good. He was learning something, and so was I. But I found it impossible to put the aid back in place. After considerable fumbling I became fearful that I might drop the fragile charm and destroy it. I gave up and succeeded in restoring it to its box. In the meantime I stood awkwardly, trying to keep my balance on the shifting floor of the subway car. That man on my right, intrigued, continued to gawk. My fumbling on this occasion taught me an important lesson, a forerunner of many that would later occur. I realized that I had to learn to endure the gawking of strangers who had noticed the contraption around my ear.

Impulsively, I made plans to launch a campaign to change people's attitudes by my own bold example. First I would practice simply telling a man that I was having difficulty understanding his words because I have some loss of hearing. After I had become accustomed to wearing the hearing aid I would take the next step and call attention to it when I could appropriately do so during a conversation. Some day, I promised myself, I would find others willing to join me in promoting widespread acceptance of hearing aids among the general public.

One day, after I had returned to my job refreshed by a spring vacation at a rustic country resort, I greeted a colleague who had stopped by my office to welcome me back. Deliberately and perhaps too abruptly, I made a comment owning up to the problem of my hearing. "I feel so rested and healthy after my vacation," I remarked, "even my hearing seems to have improved."

"Yes," he said, nodding, and added, to my astonishment, "We've all noticed." We? So they had known. How long? But not a word had leaked to me!

Suddenly, and for the first time, a memory came to me of a day at a children's camp where I had been working as a counselor along with several other college freshmen. We were sprawled on the carpeted floor of the lounge after hours, relieving our tensions by gossiping about the supervisory staff. One of the girls lowered her voice and described a misunderstanding she had had with Amanda, the head counselor, that morning. One of the boys circled his arms around his propped-up knees and leaned forward to whisper a secret. "Did you notice," he said with significant emphasis, "that Amanda wears a hearing aid?"

There was a moment of silence, and then someone asked,

"Are you *sure?* How would you know, with that curly hair covering her ears?"

"I'm sure, *I'm telling you.* I watched her fussing with her hair one day. I saw her take it off, run a comb behind her ear and put it back on."

Someone else said, "Maybe she doesn't wear it all the time, because it seems to me she hears better some days."

I added my contribution to confirm the revelation. "Once when we were getting together in the mess hall on a very cloudy day, I remember she asked me, 'On a day like this when it looks like rain, the noise in this big room is awful. The weather seems to affect my ears. Have you noticed? Do you feel it?' "

I didn't answer her. It was a new idea. I hadn't been aware of any difference in acoustics due to air pressure. (Today I would have noticed.)

As I now recalled that evening, it was clear to me that we had coalesced into a friendly huddle, separate from Amanda, because we were sharing knowledge of her secret. I carried the impression thereafter that this august staff person was flawed, different, not like the rest of us.

That gossip session happened a long time ago. Granted, such a situation would surely not affect me so profoundly today, but because I had become so vulnerable, the memory attached itself to my immediate apprehension. Since my colleagues, who were also my friends, had indeed been talking about me, what exactly had they been saying? Did my hearing problem affect my reputation as a competent staff member? Was I diminished as a person? The keenest emotion I felt was anger—unreasonable anger at them for shielding me and at myself because I was confused about the way I had reacted. I had projected the attitude of those young counselors, standing aloof from Amanda, to accommodate my own sense of being left out. I saw that I was thinking now about them versus me. My bold decision to tell everybody about my hearing aid had been thrown into high relief.

I had not yet established the habit of wearing my hearing aid. I used it intermittently, in certain situations when I knew that a failure to hear would be a serious handicap, but I did feel safer, having it as a resource, and I carried it with me at all times. By this time I was also becoming aware of its drawbacks. Its chief advantage, that it amplified sound, was also its glaring defect for anyone with nerve deafness, a condition which causes one to experience sudden bursts of loudness beyond anything that a person with normal hearing would hear. I needed the amplification in order to hear on the levels at which my hearing was defective, but I could not tolerate the occasional shocks of unwanted loudness.

I phoned Ashley Baker at the New York League to ask what to do about the loudness. "It's not going to harm you," she said. "It would have to be much louder to do any further damage, but you can't avoid it. Perhaps you're turning the power up too high. Keep practicing, until you get to know how to modify the amplification just enough and not too much. But be sure you wear it—wear it *all the time.*"

In the shelter of my home, I kept fiddling with it, making adjustments to comply with the rise and fall of any sound I needed to hear. I listened to the television with my finger working the power switch constantly, because the background music, the commercials, and other programmed sounds caused a succession of blasts that impeded comprehension. On the telephone, a slight rise in the voice of a caller making some emphatic statement banged against my eardrum. I lacked the mechanical expertise to adjust the power properly, and I also lacked the patience to keep trying.

In all the current magazine articles, in newspaper columns, and in glowing advertisements, I had read: "With our new technology now there is a hearing aid that can help you to hear even if you have nerve deafness." Nobody had warned about the shortcomings. (Perhaps they had; perhaps the warnings were stated, however obscurely, in the literature and I had glossed over them.)

I balked against wearing the aid for long stretches for other reasons. The crescent-shaped piece behind my ear never felt anchored snugly. Often it slipped down, dangling from the rubber-coated wire against the side of my head. If the mold was securely in place in my ear the aid might hang for some time before I was aware of it. Sometimes the whole contraption came away and landed on my shoulder, where I caught it before it dropped to the floor. ("Be careful not to drop it," I had been warned. "It might be damaged.") I became wary lest it fall off in the presence of other people, and I often raised my hand to check that it was still in place.

The mold in my ear presented other problems. If I kept it on for an hour or more, I had an allergic reaction to the plastic that caused itching. I phoned the dealer to ask what to do about this difficulty.

"We can change to a rubber mold," he suggested. "But I can't guarantee it will help. It probably bothers you because you're not used to it. Give it time." Fortunately I believed him. Eventually—a long time later—I noticed the itching less.

But the mold was a foreign object stuffed into my right ear. It felt like a warm earmuff, unbalanced by the cool free air that circulated around my left ear. I longed to set my ear free by ripping it out, and in fact I often did.

Alas, the honeymoon was over. I had been granted my wish, to be able to hear better, but at the same time I had new problems. I cherished my possession and was sure I would never again want to be without it, but I had a long way to go to surmount the unforeseen drawbacks.

FOUR

My First Hearing Aid

For several months I was content merely to carry the blue velvet box with me in my purse. In spite of my disenchantment I valued it as I did the diamond ring and pearl necklace in our bank vault and enjoyed knowing that I had it in my possession. Each morning I came to my office before the rest of the staff arrived, shut my door, and inserted my hearing aid. I listened with relief to the amplified thud of the box lid as I closed it. ("It's working!") I tested the aid over and over, hoping I had both parts correctly in place. I relished this quiet opening of my day alone, before sound and interaction had built up. Nestled in the springy office chair with a cup of hot coffee, I listened to the sweetly muted tones outside my closed window, softened as in a dream. Gradually there came the familiar indoor sounds, now so clearly relayed to me by my hearing aid—the click of heels, the surge of cheery morning greetings, the gurgle at the water cooler, the muffled drone of typewriters being pulled out and raised to desk level—through my closed door. I enjoyed wearing the aid for an hour or more. But ultimately the noise level rose by many decibels, and the cacophony destroyed my serenity.

I was one of the directors at the national headquarters of the YMCA, at that time located in the Wall Street area of New York City. I was the editor of the *Circulator*, the national

YMCA publication distributed to the staff directors in 1,800 local YMCAs and thirteen foreign countries and circulated among their local staffs. One of my objectives was to report the most innovative and effective programs in local YMCAs that were offered to the membership in each age group, giving enough details so that such stories would constitute a resource for adaptation in other Ys. The *Circulator* also contained reviews and descriptions of seminars, lectures, conferences, and special educational (and inspirational) courses designed by Y regional executives for the training of local staffs. These made it possible for the attending local Y directors to enhance their services to their constituencies.

To cover the field I had built up a widespread relationship with other national family agencies, family counselors, marriage therapists, social agencies, college faculties, religious organizations, behavioral scientists, and researchers in the field of applied psychology. I livened up my publication with generous insertions of material contributed by a new breed of innovators who hoped to promote personal fulfillment through nonverbal methods, using body and sense awareness. We called it a "Human Potential Movement." Its gurus included several people who were experimenting with ways to change human behavior; even these were given space in my publication because they represented a very popular trend in the 1960s and did in fact develop many excellent techniques that have since been adapted by responsible therapists and counselors. I now see many of their programs listed as courses in college and university catalogs and in church programs to serve the religious community. I learned enough, through critical participation in programs, by consulting with program leaders, and from studying their materials, to extract the information that would be useful to Y program staffs who read the *Circulator*.

While I worked alone in my office, there was no need for the amplification of the aid, and I usually removed it to restore quiet in my environment. (I had put up a sign on my door, "Please come in. It's open.") Occasionally I preferred to keep the door open so as not to feel cut off—or shut out! Someone with a question might stand at the threshold or would enter to consult me or just to invite me to a coffee break. If the visitor failed to speak a few decibels above the background clatter, I wished I had had the time to reinsert my hearing aid. But even on occasions when I was wearing it, certain sounds were amplified beyond my tolerance level, and a comment or question just hung in the air until the visitor repeated it or simply gave up and departed.

Ashley Baker had urged me to call her if I had any problems, as did the dealer. I called both and received the same advice: "You're probably not using your aid enough. You'll never get adjusted to the way it sounds with background interference if you don't wear it *all the time*. The loud noise won't bother you as much, and you'll learn to listen attentively so that you'll be less conscious of the distortions."

In one kind of situation my aid was truly helpful. I often attended conferences in large rooms or meetings held in auditoriums with a speaker standing before a podium. On these occasions I blessed the scientists who had developed this wonder-working invention that rescued me from a sea of confusion. If the acoustics were adequate, and the audience quietly attentive, I marveled at the clarity of the speaker's words, which sped through the microphone to my hearing aid. I came to revel in the aid's snug presence in my ear.

I was using my hearing aid as anyone might use a walking stick on a dangerous country road—only when I knew I would otherwise be in serious trouble. Often a whole week would go by without my opening the box in my purse. But I had given up on the aid as an everyday tool. It was hard to convince Lou that, when I wore it, as he kept badgering me to do, I was disturbed even by sounds in the next room—

sounds he was not able to hear. These unwanted sounds, as is usual with nerve deafness, seemed to me as loud as, or louder than, those nearby. The mishmash of distorted noise outweighed the advantages of amplification, and I opted to be completely free of the nuisance. I had little opportunity to learn to manage the aid's power, to learn new ways of listening so as to surmount the harassment of my noise intolerance. I was not combining the benefits of amplification with closer attention to lips, eyes, and gestures so that even the distorted sounds would become more intelligible. (Years would pass before research technologists made any progress in reducing some background noise.)

I continued to feel insecure during one-to-one encounters with office colleagues and worried about lapses in interpretation. Who knows how many times my coworkers had been puzzled by an irrelevant response? All the offices were noisy during the greater part of each day with the buildup of activity. I was always hesitant to ask speakers to repeat themselves. ("You've done that; don't try it again.") I had other worries; what would I do if the battery suddenly went dead? What if it slipped from behind my ear in their presence? (I was still using the two-part model with the aid behind my ear, attached to a tube that connected with the mold in my ear.)

I had not yet been willing to show people my hearing aid. ("But you promised!") The real trial by fire came on staff meeting days, which occurred once a month in a conference room large enough to allow tables to be fitted together to seat as many as twenty people. Usually we had a dozen in attendance, so that our seating arrangement might cover an area about sixteen feet in length and about five or six feet across. Since my hearing threshold at the time was a distance of six feet, I was still able to avoid using the aid. I was able to manage (or at least I hoped to do so) as long as there was no particular drawback. But so often there was! If a new arrival or an office messenger opened a door and shut it noisily, I lost a few words. If people coughed or blew their noses, or if someone near me had a nervous quirk of clicking a pen open and shut, I missed a few more. If a trailer truck passed outside, I was in dire trouble. How grateful I was when someone else asked the group's permission to shut the windows. (Never would I be the one!)

Thus it followed, day after day, that as the morning began I ritually asked myself: is this a day to wear my hearing aid, or dare I trust to luck and keep it hidden?

I reviewed the events that were coming up: X was due back from his field assignment of visiting the Far West cluster of YMCAs. Was this the morning he would arrive, bringing back information that I should report in the *Circulator*? He might just walk into my office for a preliminary chat about it. His was the voice that gave me my biggest problem. X possessed a penetrating intellect, a mind with a razor edge, and the muted voice of the introvert he was. His gestures, even his facial expressions, were contained. His thin lips just barely parted over a tight mouth as he spoke. A perpetual tiny smile crinkled the skin around his eyes, but his speech remained a total monotone. He could be delivering a rare treasure of new information without increasing the sound of his voice by a decibel. As the significance of his statement reached me, delayed by a fraction of a second because of the failure of nerve fibers to deliver the words to my brain, I became stiffly alert to what was to follow, not quite sure I had heard it all and correctly. If I was wearing the hearing aid and the door was closed, I was in clover. If I had not inserted it that morning, I suffered remorse. Sometimes he seemed to be studying my face intently. Was he wondering whether I had heard him?

A staff meeting that lasted all day was problematic. Mr. X was usually conscientious about arranging his schedule so as not to miss it. The younger men with the least seniority spoke with a low-keyed diffidence before this group of mixed hierarchy. I could not erase from my awareness a mental image of Tom, that brilliant former member of the staff, now retired, and his antics shortly before he retired, when his fingers never left the little black box that hung on his chest connected by a wire to his ears. After we began to question how much he was hearing, he was no longer as vital a participant on our team. Without meaning to do so, we had distanced him. What will happen, I thought, when I tell them about my own mechanical device?

After experiencing the help that an aid might give me, I became more sensitive to my handicap, but I dreaded having the aid in my ear for a stretch of five or six hours. For more than a decade, and especially before my hearing had begun to fail, I enjoyed staff meetings. They provided a rich resource of material that I would then follow up for report and discussion in the next issue of the *Circulator*. Besides, I was grateful to have found a vocational situation that provided the most beautiful friendships anyone could hope for. I had a long-standing love affair with the whole staff, people I admired for their intellect, their spiritual qualities, their graciousness in response to criticism, and their rollicking good humor.

I recall what happened to me toward the end of one such all-day meeting with a cold sinking feeling. We had been in session for four hours before the lunch recess. Most of us rushed back to our offices to see whether anything needed attention. I phoned for a sandwich and remained at my desk, uncurling my back and stretching every muscle, pleased with how well the morning had gone without the hearing aid. But I began to feel nervous about the final two hours. How well would I do when fatigue set in? I was truly ashamed of my cowardice after having boasted to my family that I would no longer be willing to allow my handicap to remain invisible. I could hear my sisters all around me when

I was little, gesturing with their fingers as they teased, "Shame, shame, fraidy-cat."

Today, perhaps, I would tell them. I deliberately made a precise plan about how I would do it. Let it come spontaneously. After all, it won't be news to them; it will simply make it easier for all of us. They'd be glad. I would also use the opportunity to make a real test of a larger resolve; I would reveal that I now had a mission to try to change the attitude of society and lighten the burden of concealment for the millions of us with a hearing loss. I would tell them how I was planning to develop a strategy to carry out my plan.

After the short break I returned to the conference table, this time wearing my aid, and seated myself without first checking to see how close I might be to the low-voiced talkers or to the one whose lips seemed barely to part. Feeling refreshed, I was able to hear better and welcomed the sound of voices, which now seemed more resonant; it was as though I had shifted the dial on the television set to bring the world back into focus. I could feel my own voice pounding. Too loud. I lowered it quickly, to avoid seeming like an over-assertive feminist in this predominantly male group. I felt truly reunited with the staff. I discovered that I was leaning back and enjoying the comfort of my chair instead of bending forward. It was restful to be so integral a part of the group, and I was happy. Only one or two hours to go before adjournment and I felt no fatigue.

The day's ordeal was not over. It was my turn on the agenda to report and I was ready with a fair-sized contribution when I noticed that everyone seemed to be listening so intently that they were actually staring. Then it happened. Something was tickling my right cheek. I lifted my hand to brush it away and felt the slippery surface of plastic. The delicate earpiece had fallen from behind my ear and dangled from the wire. Quick as a flash, I replaced it, but I couldn't change the expressions on the faces around me. I ended my report sooner than I had intended, and the discussion resumed as though nothing unusual had occurred. I kept quiet, wondering how soon my perspiration would stain my blue silk blouse.

Why not tell them today, just after we cover the last item on the agenda? How about: "Oh, by the way, I've got this hearing aid. . . ." (show them, and smile.) I was ready to do so when paralysis seized my vocal chords—and my hearing too! I was only subliminally aware thereafter that a discussion of some last points was still in progress. Then, suddenly, I noticed the gathering of papers and shifting of chairs and realized that someone must have announced adjournment.

I left the office seething with frustration. I had not yet fully accepted the permanence of my hearing loss, but I was unaware of my resistance. Deep within me I still expected to awaken someday to an extraordinary restoration of my hearing, as though the lapse had been only temporary. If I were to acknowledge it now, the magic of such promise would dissipate. This is not an uncommon reaction. It occurs quite frequently among people with the onset of any irrevocable handicap or chronic illness relatively late in life. I had had no guidance to help me overcome my emotional block—an essential ingredient, I was later to learn, in all prognostic treatment programs.

I was gripped by resentment that this widespread impairment remained underground, whereas millions of people with poor vision could display their problem openly. Eyeglasses had become a hugely profitable industry. People ordered frames in all shapes and colors to match their costumes. The most staid conservatives could wear them with dignity; high-styled in gold, glasses sparkle with a hint of affluence. Why should I have come to expect a harmless unit tucked behind my ear to prompt uneasiness in everyone who caught sight of it?

Home was no refuge that day. It was no longer "*When* are you going to go for a hearing aid?" but "Why aren't you wearing your hearing aid?" Lou put the question to me the very moment I uttered the familiar, "What did you say?" Coming at this time the question destroyed any urge I had felt to talk about the meeting at the office. I spent the evening quietly, staring at the pages of an open book.

Whenever Lou or Susan badgered me about not wearing my aid, I went through the same narration. They seemed never to *hear* my explanation, each with their nice, good ears:

"I did have it on, you didn't even notice, but I took it off when it wasn't helping. Everything gets louder, and the words seem to get screwed up by other noises—the television, the air conditioner, even the refrigerator. I can't stand the water running in the kitchen sink. Even when you talk to me while you're rattling the pages of your newspaper, my hearing aid picks it up and I miss a few more words."

"You won't get used to it if you don't wear it."

"I will. . . . I'm trying. . . ."

No one who has not had to use a hearing aid for nerve deafness can possibly imagine how the contamination of sound seems at times. When I tried to explain, I met with indifference, impatience, or sheer boredom. Quickly there would be a change of subject in the conversation, which further embarrassed me. ("Not *my* problem.") But it *is* everyone's problem that hearing aids gather dust in people's bureau drawers.

These frank encounters occurred only with family and close friends who knew I used an aid. Several times when I offered to lend my aid to one of them for a few minutes' trial they backed away. "Look, I'll wipe off the ear mold with a cloth soaked in alcohol, so it will be perfectly sanitary." Their faces screwed up in distaste. I took the response as personal rejection. Of course, people don't normally ask to borrow a pair of crutches, either, in order to understand better how it feels to be crippled. But lameness is a sharply visible handicap; you can see what is happening. You can relate more intelligently to a lame person. Likewise, if you're communicating with a friend who is wearing a patch on one eye, you know at once the kind of problem that that person is having with diminished vision. But who can guess how the invisible hearing loss, to whatever extent it is offset by an almost invisible hearing aid, is altering perception of one's world?

One day while I was attending a wedding reception I wandered about the noisy crowded room with a glass in my hand. I felt reluctant to enter into conversation with people in separate little clusters, but I envied them and was lonely. Everywhere there was laughter. I picked up words from the repartee, but the conversation went too fast for my lagging comprehension.

I passed a group that included my husband. I savored his pleasure at being free of the responsibility of my dependence, and I flashed him a smile to let him know I was all right on my own. His eyes were sparkling as he entertained his listeners with one of his many droll stories. How I loved him at such times and enjoyed watching the pleasure he gave and received by his gift of instant friendship. Like a being out of nowhere I flitted about, determined to derive some pleasure from the joyful event. To counter my isolation I absorbed myself in each of the scenes being played out before my eyes.

Suddenly my attention was drawn to the tall, lithe figure of Evan, a young man I had known for some time. Because Evan is a behavioral psychologist as well as a friend, we had talked about my impairment. Perhaps he could rescue me from the embarrassment of my isolation if I joined him and anyone else he drew into a friendly circle. At the moment he appeared to be not too closely involved with others and was nibbling from a small dish of hors d'oeuvres. I waved to him and was rewarded with a signal of welcome and a radiant smile. I approached him with some relief. Here I would find a safe harbor. Evan motioned toward a young woman nearby to join us.

"You two should get to know each other. You both have something special to talk about."

Putting his arm around her slim waist, he introduced Billie. I was struck by a dainty quietness in her thin face. Her eyes smiled calmly. Her delicate cheeks shone smooth as silk. She greeted me with friendly interest that was comforting. Evan explained that she was more than marginally hard of hearing. I marveled at how Evan could mention it so casually in her presence. She told me she had been so impaired from the time she was twenty, which I judged was perhaps fifteen years earlier. The three of us communicated with satisfaction even in that difficult environment because we knew how, speaking slowly and enunciating clearly. Here were two people enjoying an intimacy that had broken through the limitations of a severe handicap. My perception of Evan immediately changed. He was no longer "one of them" but "one of us." He had stepped over the barrier that the world outside had become for me, and the connection was as welcome to me as a warm embrace. For Billie's sake as much as for mine, Evan asked how I was managing with my new hearing aid in the turmoil of this environment. Quickly I offered to show him.

"I'm not sure. Would you like to try it?"

Without hesitation he reached for it. He wore my aid for perhaps five minutes in that crowded room, amid all the tumult of celebration. I watched his face and vicariously felt the assault of the barrage of amplified sound. He grimaced at the shock of the sudden hullabaloo. "Here. Take it back," he begged, jerking the ear mold off and violently shaking his head as if to rid it of the rawness of the amplified sounds. "That was a long five minutes!"

"It wasn't exactly a fair test," I conceded. "This is one of the worst places to try it. I had to learn that; I turn it down now when it gets too awful."

"But if you turn it down, how do you hear me when we talk in a place like this?"

"I don't! It's catch 22. That's when I get discouraged and try doing without it. Everyone thinks I've got hold of a magic solution with this little invention. You can see it's a mixed blessing."

How I wished my family and friends would try Evan's experiment. The ordeal of becoming reconciled to the limited advantages of a hearing aid became an obsession. A constant distraction threaded through my thoughts during every activity and concern, like the dieting woman's obsession with calories. Dieting women had an advantage, however; they could talk about it—and how they did!—with laughter. They were able to chatter about their predicament, but I went underground with mine. I craved the company of anyone else who might understand my stress and might be willing to talk about it. Evan had wandered off by this time, but Billie stayed, interested and helpful, using her own experiences for illustration. I clung to the subject matter for a long time, odd as it was in the midst of a wedding reception; I was totally oblivious to the contrast between topic and occasion. Reluctantly I at last let Billie rejoin Evan. I moved away to the refreshment table, where it would be easy to carry on idle conversation with any stranger.

Several weeks later my husband and I enrolled for a week's holiday at Bucknell University. We were participating in an "elderhostel," a vacation program for people over fifty-five that is offered on college campuses around the country. Courses are provided on the college level by college faculty—a treat for people who, like myself, wished to extend our education with the accrued wisdom of adulthood. Lou and I had chosen Bucknell because the course featured a uniquely powerful telescope for which Bucknell was then famous. Our lecturer, a ruddy young professor who looked as though he spent his leisure hours on a ski run, led us to a flight of stairs. He took them two at a time to the top of the building where the telescope was set up and called down to us to follow. There we were privileged to have a startlingly intimate view of the moon. I was astonished by its closeness; the craggy surface seemed no more than ten feet away.

One at a time we took turns at the telescope while the professor kept adjusting the focus on jagged shapes and scratches and on large and small craters. Each viewer emerged, gasping with surprise. The group's mood became spiritual. I had positioned myself closest to our mentor, as I had learned to do in every classroom situation. Suddenly I made a discovery that held me transfixed. His right ear was plugged with an ear mold, but there were no tubes attached. He was using an in-the-ear hearing aid! I had only recently learned, after all the fanfare about President Reagan's aids, that this new type was being widely marketed. Ads for the new invention were appearing in the popular media, but the sober articles I studied in professional publications cautioned the gullible public against rushing out prematurely to acquire it. "It's not for everyone."

I watched our zealous lecturer's face for clues as to how well he was hearing, for he often had to interrupt his talk to field questions from all parts of the room. The drama of his illuminating discourse reached me in a fog because of my preoccupation with his inner-ear device. He was ready with a quick response to each question and never once asked for a repetition, nor did he reveal any failure to hear correctly. *His* hearing aid worked fine for him. What was wrong with mine—or with me?

The scheduled session over, participants huddled around the professor begging for encores, for answers to more questions. I pictured myself raising the ones that had priority for me. How do you like wearing your aid? How long have you had it? How long does it take to get used to it? Were you able to hear everything during the session today? Did you use to use the behind-the-ear type? Is this doing a better job? Do your students notice? Does anyone ever mention it to you? Did you use an aid when they hired you to teach? And so on and on. The questions swarmed in my head, for I was overcome with awe of a hearing-impaired faculty person of his scholarly stature who could function competently among his colleagues in a university. I imagined the reaction of the professor and the class if I broke through their clamor for moon facts with my own irrelevant questions.

I judged from the man's youthful appearance that his was not the presbycusis common in the elderly. I wondered whether the new gadget in his ear would do any more for me than the device with which I had struggled so long. At least I had come to understand its limitations. Though I used it irregularly, it had become my security blanket, like the stuffed animals that children carry around, sometimes hugging them, sometimes using them to vent anger. My attitude toward it was ambivalent. Every day I went through the motions—hearing aid in and out of the blue velvet box, on and off my ear—hour by hour and always stealthily. On days when I was not scheduled to attend meetings or conferences, I sometimes left it at home, challenging my growing skill in speechreading against the background noises during one-to-one encounters. I was getting better at adjusting the volume of sound appropriately. I had even ventured to increase the number of acquaintances with whom I shared my secret. I was slowly building a support group with whose members I could feel at ease.

Often a memory flashes through my mind, sudden and irrelevant, to brighten the hour. They keep coming back, these pleasant little vignettes. There's one I enjoy over and over, about how I celebrated a birthday after my hearing loss.

"Make a wish," someone said as I stood over the candlelit cake, enjoying my party with family and friends. "But don't tell," I was warned. "If you tell, it won't come true."

I drew a deep breath over the glowing candles, then was startled by the spontaneous emergence of my deepest longing. A prayer in my head throbbed, "I wish to meet at least one other person who is hard of hearing like me, and we stay together with our secret and become real friends."

It seemed a weird request, because my life was rich in friendships. But a hearing loss breeds fear of desertion. Where did I belong? Merely making that wish seemed to spark a promise. Now I understood the song, "Wishing will make it so." Day after day, on some strange, less than conscious level, I was conducting a quest. I longed for people with whom to share the part of me that had become disconnected. I was absorbed in a search of strangers' ears, looking to see if any held an earmold.

Shortly after the day of my birthday wish, I made plans to attend a program being offered not too far from headquarters on problems confronting stepchildren and stepparents after remarriage. The subject interested me particularly because the program directors in the YMCAs were becoming aware of new problems in the families among their membership. There was to be a week's training seminar for those involved in helping divorced parents with second marriages to understand and manage the complications in their new relationships. It was sponsored by a team of marriage counselors working in family life organizations who had experienced an increased number of requests for help. I enjoyed such opportunities and assiduously made notes to tell

YMCA staff how to incorporate helpful materials in their own regional training sessions. Usually they engaged outside professional consultants in family life or education.

I arrived on the opening day of the program, carrying my hearing aid in my purse for use only if I had any difficulty. As I assessed the room—its size and the acoustics—I noticed that the windows were all closed. As the participants arrived one by one, I tried to gauge the quality of each person's voice. There was a good deal of movement in the room as people went about greeting each other. Comfortable chairs were being shoved into places, but I judged that the seating arrangement would not present a problem. I decided I would not need my hearing aid and kept it in my purse.

As we were about to begin the session I chose a seat with my back to the window so that sun or bright light would not obstruct my view of people's faces around the oval in which we were seating ourselves. What happened thereafter is vivid in my memory. I cannot even dimly recall who led the workshop and delivered the introductory address, for I had become curious about the woman on my right.

In my mind's eye I see her dress, a simple beige sheath, and her permed hair framing a round, pleasant face. She is rummaging through a floppy canvas bag. With the excessive curiosity of an editor I follow her movements as she draws from the hodgepodge of a careerist's collectibles a familiar-looking velvet box. She opens it cautiously with a glance around the room and removes *two* hearing aids. *This* woman will be my companion for the day.

As she proceeded to insert the aids, she noticed my gaze. With some hesitation she explained sheepishly, "This is my first day. I don't know yet how these things are going to work for me."

"Me too," I said, with some excitement, although more than a year had gone by since I first acquired my aid; I still used it so infrequently that I considered it "new." I opened my purse and showed her my aid, whereupon her face brightened in an attractive smile. She began to talk about her hearing problem with animation and twinkling candor, and we immediately became close friends. Seated beside such a cordial ally, I felt empowered to endure my own aid. I followed her example and boldly inserted it in my ear without looking to see who was watching. We both thirsted for the details of each other's experience and burst into a rapid-fire exchange of questions. Fortunately the conductor of the workshop had had to interrupt his opening address while several more people arrived and chose seats.

"How long have you had yours?" "Do you take yours off a lot?" "Is it hard to get them on, when you have two?" "Did yours ever drop off and dangle around your face?" "Does it *really* help you to hear?" "Does your permanent cover it enough so people can't tell?" "Do you ever try using just one at a time?" "Did you get yours for your good ear or for the worse one?" "Do you tell people?"

We stayed close to each other for the length of the session, ate together, freshened up side by side in the large restrooms, took our twenty-minute breaks and short walks together, and said good-bye with a warm, tight hug. It was an unforgettable moment in my life.

Another fellow sufferer who will remain nameless set a memorable example for me at an evening performance of *Man of La Mancha.* Lou and I had good seats in the center section of the orchestra, an extravagance. I curiously surveyed the crowd and noticed a happy young couple settling down in the row in front of us. The man helped his companion remove her jacket, then reached into his pocket and, without stopping his conversation, withdrew a small box. Out of it he produced a familiar two-part model of a hearing aid. Instantly I felt that wonderful kinship, this time with a total stranger. He affixed his aid deftly and effortlessly, while

I still performed this process clumsily, noticeably. During the entire play, my attention strayed from the stage to the couple in front of me. His head turned often toward the woman as he whispered to her. Each time I had a glimpse of the aid, visible in profile, and more of his face. He looked so comfortable, so happy, so unashamed. Since he was probably less than forty years old, he may have had a condition that started early in life, perhaps at twenty or when he was even younger, and was apparently thoroughly accustomed to using an aid. Would I perhaps someday be as free?

During intermission Lou asked, "What have you been looking at down there?"

"That couple sitting in front of us. Didn't you notice? He has a hearing aid. I watched him take it out of his pocket and put it on when they arrived."

"They look happy, don't they?" Lou observed. "Obviously in love. Being hard of hearing didn't slow down their romance—probably enhances it." (Was he telling me something?)

On the way out to our parked car he asked, "How was it?"

"Wonderful! Much better with my hearing aid." I skipped a few steps.

There was a light snow, but the wind was sharp. I welcomed its sting as we twisted and turned to ease our way through the departing crowd. The crystal flakes were soaking a ticket stuck on our windshield. We had parked on the wrong side of the street. With a shrug Lou stuffed it in his pocket. Who cares about a parking violation when I'd just leaped over a hurdle!

One day I observed that my batteries were going dead more often.

"Could be because you're using them more now," Lou suggested. Gradually I was becoming reconciled.

"It takes a long time, I guess. Or maybe" (dark terror) "my hearing is getting worse and I can't do without it any-more."

"Nonsense," said Lou. "If you need to convince your-self, why not get another hearing test? It's been almost two years."

FIVE

In-the-Ear and Binaural Hearing Aids

The ads in all the news media about the new in-the-ear aid ("Now you can hear even with nerve deafness") were proliferating. During an overnight stay at a hospital for minor surgery, I learned that the audiology department could test my hearing. I had some misgivings about making an appointment; I was afraid of what a new test would find. But as I was leaving the hospital carrying the routine discharge form, I discovered that my feet had led me straight to the audiologist's office. The male audiologist at the hospital, unlike Ashley Baker, was a stony automaton who performed the now-familiar testing routines mechanically. I followed his instructions dutifully, trying to match his cool indifference by tuning out my anxiety. I thought I was in fine fettle, stacking up high marks with all the right answers. When it was over I held my breath while he busied himself maddeningly, straightening out and clearing away all his paraphernalia. I tried to bridge the chasm of his nonchalance with a wan smile and clever quips, but he was remote. As he studied the results on the audiogram, I saw only the black bushy swirls on the back of his head.

"You have a 'moderate' hearing loss," said the voice.

"It was 'mild' the last time," I said, very timidly. "That means it's worse, doesn't it?" Through the pounding in my ears I strained to hear his next comment.

"Not exactly. Because I see your discrimination is unusual for a person of your age with a hearing impairment. It's almost normal. That means your hearing is more functional than the tests would indicate."

"Discrimination"—that vague term again, so inadequately discussed in the material I had read, although for me it apparently represented a lifeline to the future.

"You should be using your hearing aid more." (How did he know?) "Put it on in the morning and leave it on throughout the day."

"I've never done that. There are so many times when I can get along well without it. It depends on where I am. Why should I go around with this earmuff on my right ear if I don't need it? It's so uncomfortable."

"You've got to get used to it. Don't just rely on your discrimination. Your hearing will deteriorate faster if you don't give it the help of a hearing aid."

"What do you think of that new in-the-ear aid they've been advertising?"

"The reports indicate it works well for some. It's not for everybody. You'd have to try it yourself."

The simple surgical procedure that I had undergone in the hospital had had no unpleasant effect, but I felt weak and was trembling when I left the building. I was aware of two resolves: I would switch to an in-the-ear aid, and I would learn more about how to preserve my high score in discrimination.

Hearing aids are expensive. I had to overcome some resistance because of the money I had invested in my first aid, a two-part model. A friend told me about her mother's recent purchase of an in-the-ear aid from a dealer in a nearby New Jersey town, a short drive from our home in Teaneck. He had sold her a standard name brand instrument at a markedly reduced price. Ashley Baker had advised that it sometimes proved useful to shop around. I lost no time in making the trip. The dealer, like the previous one I had used, was patient, attentive, and sensitive. He answered my questions adequately, although he spent only a moment on the subject of discrimination, as if he did not believe it worthwhile to give me too technical a response. I experienced the same frustration in reading single-page flyers prepared for the lay public.

The modestly equipped office was not impressive as a place for conducting the kind of hearing test I had had at the New York League. A licensed audiologist would have insisted on a thorough examination, which in a way accounted for my willingness to bypass such a visit. The one I received here was a brief, routine procedure. I wanted it that way! I did not want to be told again what had happened in the years since my first test. I did not dare to check it out. I was still unable to acknowledge my handicap fully and clung to the fantasy that it might not be getting worse. Perhaps this attitude explains the relief I felt at the casual attitude of the dealer; his omission of any professional discussion and his superficial testing constituted a kind of charade in which I readily participated. He was in the business of selling hearing aids; I presented myself, even ostentatiously, as merely a purchaser. All I wanted was for him to sell me a reliable article at the best price. I showed him the model I had been using and asked,

"Do you think I'd do better with one of those new in-the-ear aids?"

"That's the model almost all of my customers are buying now. You can try one I keep here. It's set in a mold that I believe will not fit too badly in your ear canal."

He placed it in my ear in less than two seconds.

"Adjust the volume yourself, and let me know how it feels."

I was enchanted by the simplicity of the device. His speech sounds seemed to move up close. I felt his presence as though we were just now meeting each other. Suddenly he no longer seemed remote. Perhaps my own faint hearing of his words, spoken in a rather low-keyed monotone, had contributed to my first impression. I suddenly found myself wondering how much my hearing loss had cost me in terms of sheer human intimacy.

In the quiet room, free of all background distraction, I felt heady with relief. The aid embedded itself snugly in the opening and felt comfortable, as if it belonged there, so unlike the crescent-shaped piece behind my ear that had always threatened to slip off. Once again the world seemed to shift back into focus. But this time I knew, of course, that the real trial would come later when I used the aid in a more normal environment, battered with extraneous noises.

"How do you like it?" the dealer asked. His eyes filled with warm pleasure as he observed my broad grin and vigorous nod. "It will be even better when I have it installed in your own ear mold."

Prudently, I attempted to slow the procedure: "How much does it cost?"

He quoted a figure little more than half of what I knew was the current price of a number of well-known brands, but I had never heard of the model he had, and I told him so.

"We sell a lot of these. But if you want to make your own investigation, you might contact someone you saw in the hospital where you were tested."

"Never mind," I said impulsively. I wanted the new aid too much to endure any delay. I negotiated the purchase with the customary thirty-day trial period.

Eight years later, as I write these lines, I am still using the aid. A recent check by an audiologist confirmed that it is still in perfect condition.

Two weeks after my initial visit I had the rapture of possessing this new device. It nestled so closely, so unobtrusively, so responsive, in my ear. I resolved to use it more—a resolve that I still was unable to follow, however, for reasons that would ultimately become clearer.

I need to explain here that my own experience does not necessarily indicate that the two-part model is obsolete. Types of hearing loss are numerous, and for many people such an aid is the only one that an audiologist recommends. Now that I have become more familiar with the coping techniques of the hearing impaired, I have reached the conclusion that each of us has a sense of hearing which is as unique as fingerprints. This places considerable pressure on the skill, training, and experience of an audiologist. Even intuitive ability must come into play as this specialist scrutinizes the details of a client's test results in order to render a final judgment regarding the most serviceable listening tool to recommend.

I became fond of my new hearing aid. I felt a lilt of joy whenever I thought about it during the day and whenever I awakened in the middle of the night. It had its own rich identity and became almost as dear as a pet from which I wanted never to be parted. I felt this fondness not only when it lodged cozily in my ear to burn away the fog of misty sound but even when it nested in a pocket of my purse. I had a supply of batteries in a bureau drawer, another in a jewelry box, and a few in my wallet. (I kept buying more!) I donated my two-part hearing aid to a hospital and shed the burden of all the anxieties it had kindled, from the first moments of false exaltation to the long siege of lapsed expectancy. I stopped blaming myself for having neglected to make more use of it. Now I was determined to obey the injunction to wear the new one. I was using it at least some time every day but certainly not "all the time," as so many people had urged me to do. There were two reasons. I did feel physically more comfortable without it—free and unblocked—but I also still needed to prove that I belonged to the world of normal people, the ones who could go about proudly independent of an artificial prop. As long as I could mingle in the mainstream of society without being found inadequate, I was not "a handicapped person," not even invisibly so.

I continued to feel euphoric about the good news that my score on "discrimination" had not deteriorated. But why, if it was so high, did I have the same baffling problem, especially when people who knew of my impairment persisted in raising their voices too loud? The only explanation I had been able to extract from all my reading was that a person with nerve deafness could often hear the sound of words clearly without being able to understand the meaning. It seemed to me that this statement described my own most frustrating sensation. When I asked people to repeat, they raised their voices; sometimes their features moved unnaturally as they exaggerated their enunciation. I was distracted and in further difficulty as their expressions changed; it made me nervous to see how hard they were trying while I continued to fail. This sequence of events occurred in a matter of seconds. I was afraid of what they might be feeling and thinking. Would they remember this difficulty the next time they wanted to talk to me and decide not to do so? To avoid such a situation I often pretended I had understood rather than ask for clarification. The consequences were frequently embarrassing.

(Only this morning, as I was sitting down at my desk to continue work on this book, the doorbell sounded. I opened it to see Ed, my nearest neighbor, a sunny, genial man, smiling at me. He offered me a plastic bag of huge cookies, still warm and bursting with chunks of chocolate and walnuts. He said something as I accepted the gift, which I could hear but could not understand. The import of his words didn't seem important, so I simply said, "Oh, how wonderful! Thanks so much."

He stared at me, puzzled, turned his head away as if

ready to leave, then turned and faced me again and repeated his statement, somewhat more slowly. This time I understood. His words were: "My wife baked these specially for our son who has been visiting, and he just left, forgetting to take along the bag."

I hastened to commiserate with him and his wife. In fact I even went overboard in my effort to compensate for my earlier failure to hear him. "Oh, what a shame. I'm so sorry. But thanks so much—and let me know when he visits next time. I owe him something for these."

Later I related the incident to Lou, who mollified me with a hearty guffaw. But the experience wasn't funny when it occurred. I nursed a little pain for a while thereafter, and I certainly hoped to give a better performance the next time I saw Ed.)

Why had I been loath to ask an audiologist for an explanation of the contradiction in my performance? I refrained, fearing that the question might somehow lower my excellent score in discrimination.

The reader will perhaps find this behavior, and other descriptions in my chronicle, totally irrational. Any psychologist can vouch for the fact that most people with healthy personalities also demonstrate inconsistencies in their behavior, but anyone constrained by an impairment is more likely to do so, especially while trying to keep the knowledge of the problem a secret.

Just at that time my daughter telephoned with a welcome suggestion.

"Mother, how would you like to talk to my friend Kathie? She's the coordinator of the Spartanburg County Hearing Handicapped Program. She has her degree in speech pathology and audiology."

"*Would* I? I've got a million questions I'd like to ask her."

"Okay, I'll ask her to come here some evening, and I'll call you back."

I harbored an insatiable craving to talk freely and at length with someone who knew about hearing loss and was not one of the audiologists I visited professionally. Now at last I would have the opportunity. The informality of the situation, and the impressive credentials of Kathleen McKenzie, created an unusual combination of circumstances that might finally address my need. There were so many gaps in my understanding that no amount of reading seemed to close. The authors of the many simplified books could not anticipate all the questions that each individual reader struggled with. I found that each book raised as many questions as it answered, but the technical journals to which I turned presented other dilemmas; I was baffled by the complexity of details, the diagrams, the formulas, and the unfamiliar technical jargon.

Kathie might rescue me. Like most people of my generation, no longer embroiled in the pace of a career at middle age, I had to restrain my impatience, and craving for instant attention. Kathie's working schedule covered a long day at her office, then the rush to pick up the children, one at school and one at the day care center. Next came an eight-hour shift of domestic duties balanced with time for the children's supper and bath. Through it all she juggled to accommodate the irregular hours of her husband's workday. There I was, barging in with my own consuming greed for enlightenment and sympathetic understanding. Weeks went by while I waited. When at last she called, she asked that we meet in her own home rather than at Susan's. Susan joined us, carrying a homemade key lime pie, which she deposited in Kathie's refrigerator. My attention was caught by two platinum-haired little children, a boy and a girl, prone on the living room floor, who glanced occasionally at the television screen. it was like a storybook scene with two joyful birds chirping at each other.

" 'Sesame Street' at this hour?" I asked.

"It gets taped during the day on our VCR."

The children were tumbling about on the carpeted floor, sometimes watching television, sometimes not. How casual and confident was their listening, with those young, unblemished ears! They could frolic on hands and knees all around the living room, note the arrival of adults, and pick up the "Sesame Street" dialog. They were so happy, so innocent, so carefree in their hearing. How many eons ago had I too listened to all the sounds of my world so casually?

Kathie lost no time as we seated ourselves at her large kitchen table. I noticed at once that she maintained an even tone and adjusted her speech in volume, pace, and pronunciation so well that I almost forgot that I had a hearing loss. Apparently she had heard from Susan that I was reluctant to increase the hours I spent wearing my hearing aid, for she launched at once into an admonition that I must wear it constantly or I would never grow accustomed to it and would lose its numerous advantages, some quite subtle. Wearing it was important, she said, "especially if you want to keep up your good score on discrimination." She then gave me an abridged description of discrimination which I paraphrase here.

"You hear sound, but that's not the same as total hearing. You need to understand the words you're hearing, so for conversation you require a more acute kind of hearing that involves the higher hearing centers of the brain. Poor discrimination indicates a particular kind of deafness we call "word deafness." A person can have serious word deafness even with only a slight loss of hearing and vice versa. The audiologist uses the microphone speech circuit of an audiometer to measure the ability to understand the words. A normal ear will report correctly a certain percentage of the words during the test, using a standardized list. With a moderate hearing loss, such as you were told you have, you should be able to repeat correctly 60 to 70 percent of the words on the test. I see from your audiogram that you were able to repeat 85 percent of the words in the test on one ear and 90 percent in the test on the other. That's terrific. You're lucky. It means that when there's no background noise, you can converse almost as comfortably as anyone with a person standing within six feet of you. That's about as good as anyone with only a mild hearing loss."

"But I don't."

"That's because of the peripheral sounds you're picking up that get in the way. Do you find that people seem to be shouting a lot?"

"All the time. It's bang, bang, bang all day long when I wear my hearing aid."

"That may be because of a problem you have in your noise tolerance level. The audiologist's copy of your audiogram here didn't include the information about your tolerance level, but it would probably show that you have a very low threshold of tolerance for sound. That means that there is a very little distance between the point at which the sound you hear seems just loud enough and the sound that is suddenly too loud for comfort. As soon as you hit that point of amplification, the loudness is so extreme that it interferes with your ability to hear accurately; that's when any background noise takes over. You're a victim of a good deal of distortion, which makes it harder and harder to understand what you're listening to. At that point, your high discrimination score can't benefit you much."

"So what can I do?"

"Try to keep the volume on your hearing aid as low as possible, even if it means missing a few words. If you wear your aid all day long, you'll get practice in doing that. And of course, as much as possible, stay where there's the least interference from background noise."

"Isn't there something they can do to manufacture a hearing aid that eliminates background noise?"

"They're working at it. It's the next step in hearing aid technology. In a few years, I believe, you'll be able to get a hearing aid that will do better with this problem. They've already been successful in eliminating background noise from devices that are being manufactured for other listening situations, so I'm pretty optimistic about this."

A sudden burst of hope filled me with a new sense of the gift of life, even at my age. I could just barely hear the children in the next room, but I thought about how different the world would seem when technology had licked the problem of background interference totally.

"The kids must be getting sleepy," I said, self-consciously shifting the focus of attention from myself.

"Oh, don't worry about them. They love it when I let them stay up, even if their eyelids are sticking together. They sleep better afterwards, so it works out."

Susan was busy guiding a spatula around the crusty edges of the pie.

"Coffee's ready," she announced.

I hugged them both, feeling comforted and secure. I had an image of the astronauts hopping about on the moon. Surely there would be progress on the planet Earth for me too; something would be invented to keep pace with the deterioration that stalked my aging ears.

As my tongue cooled around the tart sweetness of lime, I was startled by a terrible wish to cry with relief. To be hard of hearing was not the worst thing that could have happened. Susan's loving concern, her busy friend's total involvement for more than an hour with my need, seemed so much to be grateful for. Besides, I began at once to pay more attention to all the sounds I could hear: the slight clink of forks on the porcelain plates, the movement of chairs as Susan and Kathie rose to gather up the dishes, then Kathie's footsteps in the next room when she lifted her two pajama-clad children off the floor and sent them to bed. Every sound

I was able to hear testified to my continued ability to get along. I finished my coffee in deep gulps and, when Kathie returned, settled back for the encouraging minilecture she delivered in the modulated speech she had trained herself to use.

"Actually, you hear remarkably well for anyone with your degree of loss."

"How come?"

"You've picked up a few tricks—the kinds of things we stress in our classes in auditory training and speechreading."

Susan interjected, "I'm not surprised. My mother works hard when she's into self-improvement."

As I was leaving, Kathie lent me some books. I was able to follow the texts more easily after that evening. I've summarized some of the information below.

While it is true, as most people assume when speaking to hearing-impaired people, that a slight increase in the level of sound may improve comprehension, there are diminishing returns beyond a certain point. Thereafter any increase will increase distortion, retarding comprehension for a second or two and sometimes eliminating it altogether.

Since listeners are never in control of the level of sound that reaches their ears, or of the pace of the speaker's words in the course of communication, they are constantly subjected to fluctuations in the ability to understand. They may catch the meaning of the first sentence; then, if the speaker raises her voice with enthusiasm, or increases the speed of her sentences, or speaks louder for emphasis, or raises her voice to be heard above noise in the environment, the listeners' comprehension scores are lowered. You can imagine the confusion that this variation in understanding may cause—on the listeners' part and also on the part of the speaker, who cannot gauge the degree to which her words are being correctly received. Often the speaker betrays her annoyance, even anger, when she is misunderstood and is constantly asked to repeat. For this reason (and others) she may sometimes be heard to remark, "She hears what she wants to hear. If she doesn't like what I'm saying, she tunes me out."

Hearing loss in the elderly, as I've said elsewhere, is caused largely by a defect in the inner ear or along the nerve pathway from the inner ear to the brain stem, where the deficiency interrupts the process of sound transmission, rendering it exasperatingly less intelligible. Much research has gone into the designing of tests to determine the listener's discrimination score, which indicates how much this process has failed to carry through its intended mission. Most audiologists use a number of standard words lists; a few also use sentences to measure the listener's "word identification" ability. Failure to identify a word is often due to difficulty in recognizing the distinction between many of the consonants, such as k, f, and s. These letters generate the "high frequency" of short, rapid sound waves. You can test this characteristic yourself by comparing the intensify (loudness) of the sound when you say these consonants with the loudness when you say the vowel sounds o or u. Thus people with this type of difficulty would be likely to confuse words such as "cape," "safe," and "face." This confusion would reduce their ability to comprehend what is being said, since they would probably be able to distinguish only the vowel sound of the a. Their hearing may even be normal for the vowel sounds, which are articulated by longer and slower sound waves—that is, lower frequencies—and greater intensity. They are consequently hearing some sounds well, some only faintly, and some not at all. Possibly such mixed reception involves only a single word, since many words contain a number of syllables with both vowels and consonants.

Shouting has a negative effect because of another characteristic of sensorineural loss due to inner ear malfunction. There is a sudden abrupt increase in the sensation of loudness when sound heard is delivered at a level higher than the person's tolerance level. A person with a hearing loss of 40 decibels above normal, for example, will comfortably hear a speaker whose voice has been raised by 40 decibels or whose speech is slow and very clearly enunciated, but if the speaker's voice goes higher than this 40 decibels by only 5 more decibels, it may be received by hearing-impaired people as equivalent to a 20 decibel increase in the normal ear that has no impairment. If even more volume is applied, the noise becomes intolerable. The strain is even more evident when a background noise in the hearer's environment intrudes, as I knew from my experience in restaurants, in a group where several people are talking at the same time, or in a room when a truck passed outside the window. It was maddening one week when a stubborn cricket made its way into some corner of our apartment and chirped all day long. My new aid, for all its efficiency and responsive power, seemed further to intensify the insect's sound.

A sensorineural loss assaults hearing-impaired people with a barrage of intense noises every day whenever they are not alone. Often they are fatigued by the loudness and seek solitude. This aggravation accounted for my tendency to pluck my hearing aid off impetuously after I'd been trying unsuccessfully to make the appropriate adjustment in the volume.

The gradual change that took place in my social behavior is thus understandable. I have always found being with people stimulating. Human interaction is fascinating in its complexity. Furthermore, although I am aware that my aliveness is defined by the presence of others, I cherish the hours I spend by myself, I am always conscious of my need to rejoin the human "collective." Now, however, I must often fight an impulse to withdraw physically, or simply to tune out by picking up a book or my mending or knitting while others in the room are engaged in conversation. I tire of the television and walk out of the room in the middle of a program to which others are listening intently. I have expressed the reason for my sudden social withdrawal only to my husband, for I dread saying anything that will make others more conscious of my handicap. I often disguise my qualms about being seen as unfriendly—as a loner—by adjusting my features with a meaningless smile that in no way relates to the cloud of loneliness in which I am immersed.

"You've got to accept the loudness when it occurs," Kathie had kept repeating. "You can't go on fiddling around with the volume, turning it up and down, because volume keeps changing minute by minute."

"But I'm worried that all that loud noise will injure my ears even further. Don't they always tell us about how teenagers are ruining their hearing with rock music?"

"That's true, but most of the time the additional intensity that you experience isn't bad enough to be dangerous. I'm not talking about the grinding of a garbage truck or a blowout."

Susan's presence was important for her and me both. She was better able to understand how I experience meaning from the sounds I hear. I could rely on her support when we both bogged down over the inevitable communication failures. In time I regained my faith that a loss of hearing would not threaten the security of the mother-daughter relationship we valued.

By this time, I was now wrestling more successfully with my struggle to get used to the aid. Each morning I opened the velvet box and carefully performed the ritual insertion. Once I had the aid in my ear, I resisted any attempt to remove it. One day, to my delight, I discovered that this new behavior was paying off when I lifted my finger—the one I used to regulate the volume—and discovered that I had not yet put the aid on. The gesture had become so automatic that I had actually resorted to it before inserting the aid. At last I had overcome the sensation that something foreign was clogging my ear; I was no longer conscious of the difference when it was not there. This moment came as no small triumph, for it had taken me years to become reconciled to my dependence on a counterfeit instrument to compensate for my handicap. I was also trying harder to curb my illogical fear that by wearing it "all the time"—by relying on it—I would diminish my present hearing ability.

When I was enjoying this final acceptance an ad in a newspaper caught my attention: "Free Hearing Test!" Of course I kept seeing such ads, but I had always resisted the temptation to respond. This time, though, my attention was held by a paragraph under the bold headline in which the advertiser both reminded the reader that hearing aids should be checked annually and offered to perform this service. My in-the-ear aid was now three years old and had never been checked. I continued to study the full text of the ad and wondered whether my aid might need some sort of adjustment Perhaps there had been a change in the dimension of the fleshy cavity of my ear so that the mold did not lodge there as snugly as it once had. Or perhaps the little flap that shut off the sound had loosened slightly. I had no way of telling, as I had come to rely on it and accepted its limitations. Impulsively I phoned for an appointment, suppressing an awareness that the ad did not mention a licensed audiologist in connection with the test. I had no intention of buying a new aid, so why not just have the one I was using checked?

The office I entered was professionally impressive. A television was turned low in the quiet waiting room. There were books and pamphlets on little tables beside comfortably padded chairs and a warm soothing light overhead. I noted especially several issues of a little magazine with its contents listed on its cover: articles that were spiritual and inspirational. I stepped softly across the carpeted floor and approached the entrance to an adjoining section where a receptionist sat at a desk surrounded by components of a computer, a couple of telephones, and various electronic devices which she seemed to be manipulating with admirable composure. She greeted me cordially and engaged me in the customary preliminary dialogue for biographical information, which she recorded on a form. Then she lifted the phone to speak to the dealer in an adjoining room, asking him how long I would need to wait. The whole procedure was cleanly orchestrated. I felt as though I had entered a cloister and could no longer withdraw.

Ten minutes later a faultlessly groomed young man emerged. I watched him bid a friendly farewell to the previous customer. He then moved across the room to me and shook my hand, introducing himself with a winning smile. His demeanor inspired trust; I immediately felt that I would be treated with competence and sensitivity. I believed, and still do, that he was motivated by a sincere respect for the service of his calling. Later, I learned that he had a good reputation which reflected both his knowledge and a record of service to his clients. In contrast, the sales tactics of some hearing aid specialists do not always speak well for the quality of their performance, especially if there is to be an ongoing relationship with the purchaser. If you are tempted to respond, as I did, to the offer of a free hearing test, it is wise to be wary and prepared to resist a hard sell.

I explained to Mr. X that I had come only to have my hearing aid checked, that I had used it for three years, and that I expected to pay for the service.

"When did you last have a hearing test?" he persisted, ignoring my request.

"I haven't had one since I got this aid."

"Well, then," he proceeded, his bright eyes aflash, "you should let me test you first. Do you have a record of your previous test?" He pointed to the small booklet in my hand, which I had brought along because it contained a description of my aid. He turned to the last page, which I had never bothered to study because it displayed a tiny graph that was meaningless to me.

"Here it is," he said. He examined the lines in red and blue on the graph. "It says you have a moderate loss in your right ear; your left is better—a mild loss."

"That's right," I said meekly.

"I'll test you today and see if there's been a change."

I was frightened. I did not want to find out, but there I was, stuck. The test he administered seemed brief and superficial, compared with the one I had received at the New York League. I had an uneasy feeling that I was being rushed so that I would have no time to protest. Mr. X entered some additional scratches on the same graph in the booklet to show me how things had changed.

"Your right ear is the same." I gripped the arms of the chair, swallowing. "The left ear is not as good as it was three years ago." (Could he, with his perfectly normal ear, hear the throb in my throat?)

"What you need is two aids. That will give you balanced hearing. Let me show you."

By this time I was feeling meek and defenseless, slightly dizzy but anxious to know the whole truth. In minutes he had an aid inserted in my left ear while I was wearing my own in my right ear. "How does that feel?" he asked, adding quickly, "Turn it up so you can just hear comfortably." His face expressed such delight and anticipation that I couldn't bear to disappoint him.

"Nice," I admitted sheepishly, "but my old aid is too loud."

"You can turn that one down now."

The idea seemed reasonable. He moved back into the receptionist's area and called out to me to adjust both aids so that I could hear him comfortably. He listened to me as I adjusted the sound of his own voice to several different levels, then asked me to remove his aid and note the difference. Obviously I had been getting some additional help from his instrument.

"But it makes my old aid sound too loud."

"That's because your aid has too much power. Let me tone it down a bit."

He moved with it into his laboratory and used some tool to reduce the power. Then he suggested that I test my sense of where a sound was coming from, with first one and then both hearing aids, while he moved about from room to room and produced some nonverbal noises with various objects. There was no denying that I did sense a pleasing difference, and I acknowledged it. My smile seemed to please him inordinately. (He was winning!)

"But my budget is just about recovering from this expensive outlay," I protested. "Besides, I get along okay. I really don't feel ready to start all over again."

It was impossible to discourage the exuberant Mr. X, no matter how often I repeated that I was definitely not going to buy a second aid.

"Just let me make a mold for your left ear anyhow," he persisted. "It won't cost you anything, and I'm not asking you to purchase a new hearing aid."

During this confrontation, I recalled that the pamphlets in the waiting room included a two-page leaflet describing the advantages of binaural hearing. I had skimmed through it with only mild interest, since it did not seem to concern me, but I remembered its essential message, which I paraphrase here: "It enables you to tell which direction a sound is coming from. You can also pick up more soft speech in noisy environments. You will hear better at large conferences or listening to public speeches. When you wear only one, you tend to turn it up too high, to make up for the sound you're missing from the other ear. It's like trying to correct your vision with a lens in only one eye; your hearing is likewise 'out of focus.' "

Still, I was in no mood to begin the process of reorientation to a second hearing aid, and I firmly said so.

Mr. X heard me not at all! I was feeling low, my stomach felt queasy, and I was still depressed by the news that my left ear was also affected. Weakly, I allowed him to go about the business of pushing soft, slightly warmed wax in my left ear and leaned back in the chair, powerless, as I waited for it to firm up. Because I continued to shake my head even after he removed the wax, he made another suggestion.

"Talk it over with your husband. I'll give you an appointment for next week, when you can bring him in too, and let's have him observe while you go through the binaural test of your hearing."

Lou is as vulnerable as I am in the face of such sales pitch. When I reported what had occurred, he asked, "But did he check your aid? That's what you went for, isn't it?"

"Oh—uh—of course. I almost forget. He said it seemed okay."

"Then how come you got into the business of a second aid?"

I shrugged and discovered that I had no rational answer.

"It just happened. He kept talking and explaining. And then he insisted on making a mold for my left ear."

There was a mischievous gleam in Lou's eyes. "You got caught," he teased.

"He didn't charge," I added meekly.

"Well, how did it feel, using both aids?"

"Better, I think. Still, I don't want it. It's a nuisance, having to put on two. And I'm not ready to struggle with adjusting to it all over again."

Lou was actually laughing. "Too bad. I warned you about these 'free' offers. Anyway, let's go. I want to see for myself."

"I'm *not* going to buy a second hearing aid. He was the one who chose to make a mold. There's no obligation. He said so. If you come with me, I'll be more convincing if I refuse a second aid."

"I doubt it. You just said it did make a difference. Why shouldn't you enjoy whatever benefit you can get from these mechanical gadgets?"

"It's expensive," I countered, turned off by his word "gadget."

"Don't be ridiculous. What about the quality of your life?"

By the time we rejoined Mr. X, Lou had convinced himself that I ought to go for binaural hearing. He offered no resistance when the hearing aid specialist suggested, "I'm going to make another mold of your ear today. I want to be absolutely sure you get the finest fit possible."

Now with two molds on the way to binaural hearing, we had both surrendered to his unrelenting pressure. Two weeks later I walked out of his office with a second little velvet box and half a dozen "free" batteries. I was poorer by $600.

In chapter 2, I described the role of the hearing instrument specialist, who is certified to sell aids without having the professional training of an audiologist. I indicated that the audiologist should always be seen for a thorough test and consultation. If the audiologist does not sell aids, or if you have been tested at a hearing center that does not sell aids, you will be given the name of a hearing aid dealer from whom to make your purchase, or you may be free to shop around and have your purchase checked during the trial period by your audiologist. Today, however, most audiologists do sell a variety of aids from different manufacturers.

In responding to the ad for a free hearing test, I ignored my own advice. I have no excuse for such irrational behavior. I describe this encounter for my readers because it is such a common experience.

In the quiet of the dealer's room I had been pleased with a sense of balanced sound, although I had not missed this advantage when I used only one aid. In the next few days, I found myself constantly revising my opinion about the benefit a second aid was giving me. In noisy situations I seemed to be hearing *too much* and therefore was aware of more distortion. Besides, I now had to monitor amplification from two devices. The process seemed to demand constant manipulation. I wondered what people must be thinking as I kept fussing with a finger around my ears. When the phone rang and I lifted the receiver against my left ear, I was startled by a shrill whistle that I couldn't stop until I placed the telephone receiver in precisely one spot.* Was my caller hearing a whistle too? I was still ashamed to explain to a caller that I was wearing hearing aids. Was I never to be free of the problem of whether or not to tell? Soon I dealt with the dilemma by simply removing the aid in the ear I used when I made or responded to a telephone call.

Binaural hearing revived all the sensations I had finally overcome when I tried to adjust to my first aid. In spite of the wisdom of theory, I failed to make it work for me and was especially unhappy in restaurants. Two aids seemed to double my confusion. My eyes roamed busily around the table where diners were engaged in lively conversation. As I studied the movements of their lips without divining more than an occasional word, I felt as if I were in a dream. Ultimately I quit trying to accept the second aid, although I carried it with me in its little velvet box in my purse, where it

---

*The dealer had not told me that I could purchase a hearing aid equipped with a special telephone switch, or T coil.

never failed to remind me that I had been subjected to my first experience all over again.

Two years later I visited an audiologist for a checkup and evaluation. I drew the second aid out of the box and showed it to him.

"Don't you wear it?" he asked.

"Almost never. Sometimes at a conference, if the person seated on my left talks to me in an extremely low voice, or is difficult to understand, then I use it. And sometimes if I'm seated in a restaurant where most of the noise is coming from a jolly party on my right, I turn off that aid and put on my left one. That's about it."

"Why don't you wear it all the time?"

"I can't stand the distortion. . . . It's too loud. . . . It's a nuisance to keep adjusting two instead of one. . . . I feel all buttoned up with two. . . . I miss the natural sound out of at least one ear that I still get when I don't stuff it up with an aid. . . . I don't like having people notice that I'm wearing two aids; that may give the impression my hearing is much worse than it is."

The audiologist listened intently. "That's a lot of reasons" was his laconic comment, tactful and obscure. I waited. Obligingly he helped me, smiling agreeably. "Well, it's helpful to have it. Gives you a spare."

"Exactly!" What a splendid vindication! I had occasionally suffered a moment of panic when I had to replace a worn-out battery, wondering whether the dreaded silence was caused by sudden deafness or by a defect in my aid. I pranced out of the office in a state of euphoria; the hearing "expert" had not badgered me to wear two hearing aids as I had feared he would.

Binaural hearing? Not yet. I knew, however, that the time would come.

SIX

Out of the Closet and Outward Bound

I look forward each week to Sunday morning, a time when television programming is refreshingly mature. For half a day the screen becomes a resource for me, a door to the world. I position myself as close as I need to, tune my hearing aid carefully so as not to overwhelm Lou, and relish the Sunday quiet in our home. A cluster of interviews and discussions with government officials, scientists, educators, philosophers, and a few quirky innovators are presented without the maddening intrusions of background music and sound effects. The format bypasses my impairment and transports me to the wonderful world outside.

One Sunday morning, just as I nestled down snugly in the pillowed rocker placed within three feet of the sound source, with my late breakfast coffee, the telephone rang. I rushed to answer but failed to catch the caller's name, even after it had been repeated, and felt obliged to make some excuse.

"I'm sorry. You'll have to say it louder. I'm having trouble hearing with the TV going." (Lou had already turned it off!)

Promptly a raised female voice said, "It's Janet. Don't apologize. I have trouble too when the TV's on. Especially now, because my hearing's not that good these days."

We had not heard from Janet and Scott since they had moved to Washington. I was ecstatic at the familiar sound of Janet's chatty voice. A startling admission exploded from my lips, "I'm wearing this new hearing aid." (I was still calling it "new"!)

"Really? Then I need to talk to you. I think I'm getting to that stage. You'll be able to answer a million questions for me."

Janet's frank disclosure sped through the telephone line, piercingly earnest. Same caution-to-the-winds Janet, free in her trust.

It was an absurd introduction, after a whole year. Janet and Scott were on their way back from a visit to relatives in Florida and called to arrange a stop at our new residence in Port St. Lucie, Florida, only forty miles out of the way. We had a good deal of catching up to do when they arrived. The two men retreated to the living room to manage theirs, but Janet and I chose the kitchen near the bubbling coffeepot. She set a shopping bag down on the table. It was bulging with goodies from south Florida, foods which she had been told were not available in the "boondocks" where we lived. Her hands went up to pat her bouncy hair, now a soft gray. She hitched up the tight waistband of her shorts so that it hugged her crisp white blouse.

"How well you're looking," she said, her blue eyes bright, her own round cheeks still golden from the short visit south. Her voice had a musical ring, just right for my hearing. I noticed that her smiling lips were still unmarred by those thin wrinkles of age which I always noticed in my first perusal of a face when I listened to speech.

"You don't get any older, Janet," I said.

She shrugged and dipped her hand into a brown paper bag, extracting a bun covered with powdered sugar and raisins.

"Try this one," she said, "and here's something else they told me you can't get around here."

Out came a huge bagel shiny with the patina of polished pine. She took a generous bite.

She watched me pouring coffee and pushed her chair closer to the table. "Is that the hearing aid?" she asked. Her head bobbed forward for a good look. And so began our reunion conversation on a subject of compelling interest to us both.

Janet assumed that the acquisition of a hearing aid entitled me to play the role of consultant and adviser, a role to which I later found myself repeatedly assigned by anyone who was beginning to be aware of a personal hearing loss. She proceeded to demand answers to the same questions that had originally confronted me. It was a cathartic session for me, for I felt that my own knots were being untied. As I responded to each question by drawing on my personal experiences, so fresh and vivid, I felt the burden of anxiety lifting for both of us. Our conversation became a counseling dialogue and pleasure trip. In clearing up her foggy understanding of what had been happening, I was reinforcing my own laboriously acquired acceptance.

"With all I've learned," I warned her, "there's much more I wish I knew. I can't give you all the answers. There's so much that's different for each person's type of loss, it's a puzzle. I'm only putting a few pieces in place for you. You should really see an audiologist."

She promised. (Two years later, she had not yet done so, although she still said she intended to!)

Before we walked out of the kitchen, she commented, "Really, you ought to write a book." It was a casual remark but then she added with a sudden glow lighting up her serious face, "I mean it. After all, you *are* a writer."

Instantly I felt hooked. Any writer will recognize the

trap. I demurred but feebly. "I'm no expert on the vagaries of the human ear."

"But you *are* an expert about yourself!"

It was a powerful observation. She had stroked the vulnerable writer in me. The idea was stashed away on the back burner with all my other aborted writing schemes, but this one would soon be warming up.

"It's an intriguing subject, Janet, but it overwhelms me. I never feel I've had enough answers, no matter how much I read. I've learned a lot from a few professional people I've talked to, but as soon as I leave them, their answers begin to sow the seeds for new questions that start to sprout. What boggles me is the way my emotions get mixed up in this problem of hearing loss. It goes far beyond the physical handicap. If only there were some sort of organization, or even just a group of people, that I could connect with, not just a one-time thing."

"There is! I remember some mention of it by someone I know; I'm not sure who, but it'll come to me. I'll find out and send you the information."

It is difficult for me to convey the power of this news, for I realize how casually it would be received by a normal listener. My skin tingled, my head whirled. She had afforded me a glimpse of heaven, and I could hardly bear the vagueness of her memory. During the rest of her visit that afternoon I kept reminding her of her promise to follow up. I could tell, when Lou kicked my leg once, from the way his lips screwed up and his eyes glared, that he was giving me a signal to pipe down. His gestures warned, "You're bugging her," but I was beyond control. I could not bear the possibility that she might forget.

Each day for weeks thereafter, as I pulled the mail out of our box, I suffered a letdown. A month elapsed before the letter arrived. Janet apologized for the delay and explained that she had finally tracked down the source of her information. She had already contacted the organization, giving them my name and suggested that I follow with a letter of my own. The acronym was the strange and unpronounceable SHHH, for Self Help for Hard of Hearing People, based in Bethesda, Maryland.

In answer to my letter of inquiry there arrived a fat manila envelope stuffed with quantities of printed material. It included a description of the purposes and objectives of SHHH, an application for individual membership, a list of twenty-two chapters in a number of states, largely in the eastern part of the country, and a suggestion that I contact one in Columbia, South Carolina, the chapter nearest to my home in Spartanburg.

I carried that bundle of documents around with me to reread wherever I went—in buses, in doctors' waiting rooms where I knew I'd spend hours, in the car while I waited for my husband to finish some errand. I studied each page as though I were preparing for an exam, and I began to dream of organizing a local SHHH chapter in Spartanburg, where Lou and I spend early spring through the fall months. The information also included a list of magazine articles reprinted from the bimonthly journal, *SHHH*, and a number of other reprints that could be ordered. I wanted to order them all! A sample issue of the publication was included, along with reprints of news from several local chapters about meetings and activities.

I felt that I was experiencing the thrill of early explorers discovering a new world. Howard E. Stone, the executive director of SHHH, himself hearing impaired, had launched the organization and, with the backing of others, had assembled a staff and dedicated people in other capacities who were committed to educating and improving the fate of the nation's hearing handicapped. On a final page among the enclosures was a handwritten note: "Please write us again." I felt as if a lush carpet had been spread to welcome me.

From several of Stone's articles in the SHHH journal I felt the force of the director's personality. The breezy style of his writings, educational, innovative, and inspiring, seemed trusting and intimate. Later people who knew him told me about his dedication, his passionate concern to promote understanding, increase research, and stimulate national advocacy. He spent his time and energy traveling throughout the country, speaking about the needs of the hearing handicapped: to be heard with understanding and to be granted the opportunity to renounce their secrecy and isolation. His skill in communicating to his audiences in spite of his own considerable handicap demonstrated to hundreds, later thousands of people that hearing-impaired individuals are capable of living a normal life. He spread before them the promise of technology that was already bringing them substantial gifts of listening devices, which he described and displayed in lecture halls and private homes.

Everywhere he appeared he brought hope and promise for the handicapped. He highlighted the miracles of progress, from the horse-and-buggy stage only a few decades ago, when the partially deaf, or at least those with adequate self-esteem, carried an ear trumpet into which a speaker shouted his message. Much less cumbersome was the unit later invented, which was carried in a box on the chest with a wire that transmitted the sound to the ears. (Some of the latter types, modified, are still required to alleviate many advanced conditions.) Stone has kept in close communication with medical men, engineering experts, researchers, and reporters for information about new developments. The SHHH journal heralds each step toward freedom. Many of the stories are submitted by nonprofessional contributors who convey their experiences so vividly that the writing seems to be the work of seasoned authors. For an up-to-date list of available journal articles and other published material that may be ordered, the interested reader should contact

SHHH directly. The address and phone number of SHHH appear in appendix 4.

I now realized, to my relief and surprise, that there was a large contingent of active hearing-impaired people who had been out of the closet for years! With some twenty-two local SHHH chapters in half the states of the nation, hundreds of people must have been enjoying support and help as a reward for openly acknowledging their handicap. (As of 1988 there were 230 chapters in forty-six states.) There had been no chapters, however, in areas where I had lived for the preceding few years.

I enrolled as a member at once and began receiving the journal as well as other leaflets, many of which described activities in various chapters. Some SHHH chapters, I learned, had only a small membership, perhaps a dozen people. I felt further encouraged to plan a chapter for Spartanburg. I knew at least a few people who might be induced to join me.

As the SHHH material kept coming in my mail, I found myself plunged into a new world, where people enjoyed a sense of fellowship in awareness of their common destiny. It didn't matter that I might never meet the other members personally. Here was a shelter where I could be myself honestly, without fear or guilt, where the impatience and anger of people who resented always having to "say it again" would be mitigated by a sense of community. On my night table lay a stack of back issues of the journal that I could read in the quiet. In this way I absorbed information and impressions that penetrated my dreams. I jumped out of bed each day, excited about the prospects for change. Instead of indulging in denial, secrecy, subterfuge, and isolation, I would triumph over my diffidence and be totally honest at the very start of every encounter. I could lift the millstone of my impediment with the bolder strategy that would ask other people for the understanding that would lighten my load.

As I describe this renewed determination to take up my battle against concealment, I am aware that my reader must be thinking: "But she's said all this before." I am making every effort in this book to portray what was happening over a period of years. I find it impossible to avoid such repetition, which relates to my reaffirmation of certain goals as I lived through stages of ambivalence. Though I made bold strides in openness, I was not always able to overcome feelings of humiliation and shame, and the result was backtracking. I came to recognize a rhythm in the process—fright, flight, *fight*—before each frank encounter. During these years I was also acutely alert to any changes that might be occurring in my ability to hear. At first the deterioration was barely noticeable, and I was able to deny it as I tested my reactions day by day. To announce that I had a hearing loss was easier when I regarded my condition as stable. But when I was finally forced to acknowledge that the problem was slowly worsening, I found I needed more courage to acknowledge my handicap. I needed to fight because openness was becoming a necessity.

The telephone was still my nemesis. I was now using a third style of amplification, an improvement of the first and second, which I had purchased and discarded. The amplification is built into the receiver. I can adjust the power from one to five by rotating a tiny dial. At first the device greatly improved communication. Best of all was Susan's comment. "It's such a relief, Mom. Now I can really enjoy our conversation." The improvement, alas, slowly decreased as my hearing continued to deteriorate. I tried to keep my daughter from noticing that the problem was returning. I answered the phone, shaking with apprehension when she called. I didn't want her to know how much of the message I had begun to miss again. Sometimes after saying good-bye, with my hand still clutching the receiver, I wondered, "What exactly was she saying?" I kept thinking, "Next time, tell her. You've got to tell her that the amplifier isn't that good for you anymore." (Sometimes I just hid in my study to cry.) She noticed, of course. Her conversation changed and shortened until it conveyed only the essential message.

Spurred by my SHHH connection, I finally stopped Susan in the middle of a sentence on the phone. I said, "Susan, try this: speak slower, and lower. I can't catch what you're saying when you go so fast, and with my amplifier on the phone, don't talk loud. It comes through too strong." I had to wait a minute before she continued. I trembled at her hesitation. Was she going to decide again to avoid calling me? I was relieved by her response, adjusted so that I could now hear at least a little better.

As I soaked up the information in the SHHH journals, I changed the focus of my concern. I saw that, intent as I had been on my own plight, I too needed to understand the viewpoint of others from whom I had been concealing my hearing loss. I reviewed all the familiar forms of response in the behavior of hearing people to which I was subjected. The hearing person wonders why I am slow in responding to a question, why I hesitate or look glazed and stare in silence, why I seem to be sharply studying the speaker's face. In a group, if my participation slackens, I appear to have withdrawn. They may be thinking: Is she stupid? Unfriendly? Perhaps prematurely senile? And why do I sometimes absent myself suddenly, seeking solitude, hoping they haven't noticed? My disappearance may reinforce an impression that I have changed in personality. The circular process of misunderstanding goes on, an unnecessary burden to others as well, which SHHH insists it is my own responsibility to lighten.

I had constantly to practice being more assertive. Instead of settling for fractured communication, I mended each breach by saying, "I'm sorry. I'm hard of hearing and I missed what you just said." Always this elicited a kind response and careful repetition. I was less often distressed by anger and impatience. Guilty feelings on both sides due to errors, misplaced laughter, silences, and abandonment were washing away. It seemed that the whole world was opening doors to set me free. Over and over I was touched by the instinctive decency of people. I felt that I had tapped a well of loving kindness with which all humanity is endowed. Everybody took such pleasure in helping me. Occasionally a person came to my rescue by alerting someone else in my presence. "You have to speak up. Charlotte doesn't hear so well," or "You're talking with the back of your head to Charlotte. Turn around." Whereas I would once have been shattered by this unsolicited intervention, I now understand it as sincere and caring. Magically, I was released from the humiliation of watching silent messages pass between people through raised eyebrows and shrugs of shoulders. When my morale needed a boost, I recalled the young man in the theater who had casually drawn a hearing aid out of his pocket and placed it boldly in his ear, all the while telling the woman beside him a funny story.

Now that I no longer felt as if an earmuff had been stuffed in my ear, I had lost one of my reasons for not wearing an aid. Although I knew I could no longer hide the knowledge that my hearing was getting worse, I was less intimidated, less apologetic, and strangely at peace. Sustained by so much understanding, comfort, and cooperation, I bore the burden and concern about my fate in the years ahead with newfound strength. I was at last free of self-pity.

I became aware that I could lighten the cargo of self-absorption I had borne in the years since my hearing loss had worsened. My own experience was a storehouse of information that I could use to alleviate the suffering of others and to educate the general public. During this period, when government was responding to pressure from numerous consumer organizations, there was a nationwide outcry to "mainstream" the noticeably handicapped by giving them access to areas that handicapped people had previously been unable to use. As a result, handicapped people were now starting to become mobile in society. Still, nothing had been done to help those of us who were invisibly handicapped. Thanks to the materials from SHHH, committed as the organization was to a program of public education, I had a resource and support to develop civic involvement in accordance with my goal. The literature that Self Help for Hard of Hearing People kept sending me made me constantly aware of the public support that the organization had generated for our cause. Through SHHH I also learned about other organizations with similar goals, about such specialized schools as Gallaudet University in Washington and specialized departments in many educational institutions, and about the efforts of other advocacy groups all over the United States. Things were happening at last to alert society, and I, too, was exhilarated by the realization that I, a writer, could share in the mission.

I began my campaign by submitting short articles to local newspapers which I titled "Coping with Hearing Loss." These elicited many responses by mail and telephone. One woman wrote: "Discovering that I wear a hearing aid, people speak to me as though I'm mentally deficient. Some shout at such a pitch I nearly faint from the thundering noise."

As Lou and I planned one of our occasional visits to New York, I scheduled interviews with staff at the New York League for the Hard of Hearing. The information I gathered there would form the basis for a number of new writing projects, and I expected also to learn more about the particular form that hearing loss had taken (and was taking) in my own case.

The drive to New York City never fails to thrill me. As

135

our car slows and we pay our last bridge toll, lights turn on in my head and heart. The world is all brightness. Here is home, where I was born and lived through my earliest years, through the turbulence of adolescence, and the astonishment of first love. My eyes are riveted on the familiar sights: the tall, dusty gray brick towers, the huge billboard displays of gargantuan human figures with gaping mouths and bulging eyes, the endless surge of trucks and cars, around which hurrying masses thread their way boldly, defying every "Don't Walk" signal. During the next two memorable weeks, with my hearing aid turned down to zero, I pound the pavements of my beloved homeland, heedless of the heaped-up dirt and grime, the discarded cigarette butts, slippery orange peels, and fluttering newspapers.

It's a short walk from the Twenty-third Street subway station to number seventy-one west, where the New York League for the Hard of Hearing is still offering its benevolent services. I punch the elevator button to the eighteenth floor without even checking my memory. My senses instantly shift back in time to the moment when I entered this place, blithely trusting that my life was about to be saved by a single device that would counteract my handicap at once and for all.

I sat for some ten minutes in the reception area waiting for my scheduled interviews. My eyes darted from scene to scene in the large, crowded room as I studied the faces of the very old and the very young. Here was a baby in its mother's arms with plugs in its tiny ears. Across the floor in one corner crawled a four-year-old boy, all smiles as he played with colorful wooden toys. Around his neck and resting on his little chest was a small, boxlike contraption. Some of the toys could be manipulated to make a sound, which the child greeted with more smiles and squeals. Occasionally the air was rent with a child's piercing call, accompanied always with a grin of delight and an exchange with a parent. These youngsters found pleasure and sustenance just in being able to make noise; they had been sound-starved before they received a hearing aid. They played happily in this Christmasy paradise of noise-making toys.

I examined the faces of the parents, intent on learning how they managed to endure their children's affliction. In these offices, at least, they seemed quietly, admirably resigned. Although I ached for their sorrow, I knew I was extremely lucky to possess so much—so incredibly much—of my own precious hearing.

Ruth Green, executive director of the League, arrived and greeted me with a warm smile. I remembered her face, sensitive and generous in its openness. She had been the staff psychologist I interviewed for an article entitled "Don't be Afraid of a Hearing Aid." My article had quoted her remark "The hardest people to deal with are the ones in your own family. They get angry because you don't hear." When I asked for today's interview, I had sent her a copy. In response she had commented, "It was refreshing to read your article. It's still timely, except for the cost of the hearing evaluation." She had arranged a series of four interviews with staff, beginning with herself.

Now that she was executive director, Ms. Green's comments were broader in scope. "Let me cite you some statistics. From 50 to 60 percent of all the people sixty years and over either have a hearing loss or will reach the stage of hearing impairment requiring mechanical help. But only a small percentage have acknowledged their handicap, and far fewer assume a social responsibility for improving the communication problems that affect both those who hear well and those who don't. That makes it imperative for hearing-impaired people to take the initiative in changing the attitude in society, impacting on all the official community agencies. When you travel, ask at the hotels for the assistive listening connections to your room. If they don't have them, urge them to install such equipment. They should have telephone amplifiers and light-up alerts in the rooms when the phone or doorbell rings. In the theater, ask whether the electric wiring has been installed so that hearing-impaired listeners in the audience, using their compatible personal instruments, can enjoy the play. Such systems should be universally installed, not only in theaters, but in churches, in lecture halls, in the large areas in schools and colleges. When the legal requirements were made for devices to mainstream the handicapped, ramps became obligatory not only at street curbs but at entrances, wherever only stairs had been in use. But nothing was done about mainstreaming to benefit the hearing impaired. Now we have the means; it's up to people like yourself to see that these things become mandatory.''

While she spoke, I felt overwhelmed by the responsibility her words imposed. For years I had been enmeshed in my private predicament, watching the relentless decline in my hearing with mounting fear and, on some occasions, even dread of the future. Her pronouncement, uttered with rising emphasis, reinforced my concern. It made my chest pound with the awareness that I had a job to do in the community. I could escape the entanglement, refrain from the tendency to withdrawal and isolation, and take her message—now my message—to the world outside. I was ready for the task, thanks to the guidance and stimulation that Self Help for Hard of Hearing People was giving me with the material that regularly came in my mail.

The next three interviews had been sandwiched in with heavy staff commitments. All the seats in the waiting room were now filled, and I tried to keep my assignments to reasonable limits. Barbara deLeeuw, the director of Mental Health Services, spoke about her work, which often involved three generations in the family, for the hearing loss of one person made demands on all—child, parent, grandparent, and all their friends. She cited as an example a person whose partners around the bridge table had learned to deal with his problem kindly and as easily as they dealt the cards. But to Miss deLeeuw he admitted his fear. What if he should become ill and be absent from the game and his partners should invite a substitute who had normal hearing? Would they take him back, still willing to endure the adjustments and strain imposed by his condition?

In a third interview, Joshua Gendel, director of technical services, helped me unravel the mystery of the mechanics of assistive listening devices, about which I had been reading for some time with a good deal of confusion. Like all the staff with whom I talked, beginning with the receptionist at the entrance, his method of communication made it possible for me to engage in conversation feeling completely relaxed. He spoke slowly, kept his voice evenly moderate in intensity, and maintained eye contact. Even when he rose to reach for an instrument to demonstrate its use, or to extract material from a desk or file cabinet, he turned to face me directly so that I could speechread every word.

Now came the contact which was to make this a red letter day, the reunion with Dr. Jane Madell, director of audiology, who had on her desk a client file labeled "Charlotte Himber." She opened the file and flipped through a pile of sheets dating back to 1973. They showed audiograms dotted with esoteric ink scratches, with notations scattered below and in the margins. There were crisp explanatory scrawls, mysteriously precise, in a variety of handwriting styles. I stared at this specter of my past, exposed like a disembodied spirit. I was stunned when I discovered from the earliest entry that my initial meeting at the league for the first test had occurred fourteen years earlier, that I had acquired my first hearing aid that year, that I had returned for checkups, and that my file held an audiogram recorded on each of six separate occasions, beginning with 1973 and ending with

1980. For each visit there was a detailed entry consisting of two typed sheets of copy under the paragraph headings "Background and Test Results," "Communication Characteristics," "Impressions and Recommendations."

Here was incontrovertible evidence that I had forgotten all but two of these visits, evidence too that I had received comprehensive service from staff people—audiologists, otologists, and others—on each occasion. At every visit my hearing and hearing aid had been tested and I had been counseled in managing my communication style, improving my listening skills, and achieving the greatest potential by using my aid. A record had been obtained from an audiologist, and each audiogram had been studied by Dr. Madell. Each entry included a report of discussions as to whether my right ear or my left should be the one to be fitted with a hearing aid, in accordance with the current test result. Here and there were statements about specific recommendations which I had later declined to follow. (How I wish now that I had not ignored them!)

Perhaps a psychiatrist could explain why I have remembered only two of these six visits. Was such amnesia due to my efforts to keep my hearing loss a secret even from myself, to maintain self-denial day after day? Oddly, I retained the impression that I had accepted my handicap as soon as I began receiving the services of the league, that at least with myself I had become brave and honest about the course of events, and that secrecy and denial were subterfuges to which I resorted only with the outside world.

Dr. Madell proceeded to answer a number of questions in the brief time she could spare, mindful as she was of the continual arrival of clients waiting outside her office. I had no problem hearing and understanding every word. As with the others, she maintained steady eye contact and carefully moderated her speech. I felt comforted by her sensitivity and concern. Suddenly, with a forward-directed gesture of her head, she asked, "Tell me, why aren't you wearing two hearing aids?"

I was startled by her question. Coming from one who had professionally reviewed the complete record of my case, the question embodied significant information that I had been deliberately ignoring for several years.

"I do have two," I answered feebly, "but I don't like wearing the one on my left ear because it blocks out all the naturalness of sound that I still like to hear. Besides, it seems to increase the distortion. I try it now and then, but I give up."

"*That's* your problem. You shouldn't give up. Try wearing it *all the time.* You need to get used to the way sounds come through with both hearing aids, even though they're different from the natural sounds. In your case, you ought to be using two aids."

There it was again, the admonishment I had heard for so long while I tried to adjust to my first hearing aid. I should wear it *all the time.* The statement strengthened my sense of foreboding. My hearing had indeed been markedly declining.

Back home in South Carolina one week later I received in the mail copies of the complete set of entries in my New York League file, from 1973 through 1980. Day after day I spread the sheets across my desk and struggled to interpret the results of hearing tests over a period of years. But although I had mastered the basic audiogram, I was baffled by these records full of squiggles and abbreviations. The typed pages of text attached to each chart offered tantalizing tidbits of information that was probably clearly decipherable to the staff technicians but confused me. Here and there, through the years, the word "improvement" leaped out from the comments, defying the stark fact that my hearing kept deteriorating, usually only slightly from test to test, but on one visit there was an alarming dip in the position of the circles (right ear) and crosses (left ear) on the audiograms.

I was distressed to learn that the hearing in my left ear had become worse than that in my right, for I had continued to place stock in an initial report that this was my "good ear." This ear had been fitted more recently with the second hearing aid, which I had rejected as unhelpful. I now understood that the greater loss in this ear, and not the aid, had made it more difficult to adjust to the distortion and loudness of a mechanical device, an adjustment I could accomplish only by wearing the aid, as I had been instructed, "all the time."

In the earliest reports, 1973 and 1974, I read the diagnosis, "mild to moderate" hearing loss. After 1974, the "mild" was eliminated; now it was simply "moderate." In one report from 1979, I read the words "moderately severe mixed loss in the right ear." The dreaded "severe" gave me as great a shock as a gunshot. The stark truth was painfully clear in the raw figures: "In August of 1977 . . ., the average in the right ear was 46dB. In today's evaluation [May 1979] . . ., it was 65dB." In order to hear normally, I would need to have the sound increased by 19 decibels more than had been required less than two years earlier.

The record for six months later read: "it is noted there has been a 13dB improvement in the right ear, but a 5dB decrease in the left ear." One year later, in 1980, I found the magic word "improvement" again: "There is an improvement in the left ear in speech discrimination ability over the previous evaluation."

The subject of discrimination was far more difficult for me to interpret from the notations on the charts and comments in the text, although in general it corroborated what I had finally come to understand in discussing this condition with audiologists years later. Discrimination scores were initially extremely high, between 90 and 100 percent, in a quiet room, with almost no decline over the total period through 1980. Scores in a noisy environment averaged around 65 percent year after year, however, with considerable fluctuations. The different environments explained problems with communication that I had been unable to account for during subsequent years. The audiologists whom I consulted always commented on my high scores in discrimination, but far lower discrimination scores would more accurately have described my experience in social situations, where speech sounds might be obscured by any slight peripheral noise. The ear is a complicated organ and the incidence of defect or breakdown in any one of its hundreds of parts is peculiar to the individual. Professional people are often reluctant to explain the intricate details of each client's condition. Moreover, audiologists seem to accent the positive during professional consultations, probably because the hearing-impaired person is already so apprehensive about what is happening and about what is going to happen. Always I went home after each such contact puzzled about omissions during the consultation, things about which I "was afraid to ask."

During the two-week trip to New York, Lou and I had arranged visits with sisters and brothers living in the area and with a number of friends we had known for forty to fifty years. Each reunion was a deeply nourishing encounter, and the time for farewells came too soon. The drain on our energies—Lou's as well as mine—had become greater, physically and emotionally, with the passage of each year; accordingly, we had planned a limited schedule.

I noted at the very beginning of these reunions that my hearing had deteriorated in a single year. For a while I pretended that I was hearing as well as the last time we had been together. The ruse didn't work; I was constantly being trapped in a misinterpretation that caused either good-natured laughter or a moment of puzzled silence on the part of a speaker. I decided to be sensible and explain frankly that I was having more difficulty than the year before.

During one lunch in a restaurant with Alma, who had been a friend ever since our freshman year in college, she talked about "an encyclopedia of birds"—or at least that's what I heard. I interjected enthusiastically, "You should see all the beautiful birds in Spartanburg. They visit us and sing to us and call out to each other all day long, right outside our windows."

Alma's lively chatter suddenly stopped. Lou pressed my arm.

"An encyclopedia of *words*, Charlotte, not birds."

I joined the laughter, this time without embarrassment, secure in the company of Lou and my dearest friend.

During another reunion, a friend whom I warned at once about my increased hearing loss described her efforts to communicate with an acquaintance who probably needed a hearing aid but was not willing to deal with his problem.

"I have to keep repeating and raising my voice. It's not relaxing. Who wants to bother?"

Her intention was to demonstrate her approval of my more sensible attitude. But I couldn't avoid receiving the comment as a warning. Who, indeed, "wants to bother"—with me? And what will happen next year if it gets worse?

Each good-bye saddened me. I knew in my heart how safe I would feel the next time we were together. My friends' loving patience had touched me like the warmth of an embrace. Each look, each word, and each soft gesture became a memory that I relived through the quiet hours in the car on the long ride home. I felt rich with the treasures of so much devotion, so much love everlasting, as we kept traveling south.

Each year Lou and I spend six months in Spartanburg, South Carolina, during the warmer months and the rest of the year in Port St. Lucie, Florida. As articles appeared in both communities, I became known as someone concerned about people with hearing loss. People called on the phone or approached me at social gatherings, but I noticed a striking shift in their conversation. It was not the physical handicap they wanted most to talk about but their feelings. Although they had questions to ask me, they needed to talk to someone with whom they felt free to unburden themselves. Their hearing loss had changed lives and feelings—not only their own but also those of spouses, siblings, children, friends, and even those of strangers such as a messenger who rang the doorbell. What to do? Hearing loss is a stark social handicap. These people felt overwhelmed by the difficult situations they were called upon to orchestrate. I was saddened by their distress. Many letters included personal histories. Some called me, they said, about "a friend." Wives described their frustration with husbands who kept denying that they couldn't hear. Men called to say that their wives were bugging them, although they didn't believe they had any problem. The underlying question was, "Is she right?"

Ultimately I came to regard myself as a spokesperson for hearing-impaired people in each of the two communities. As I continued in this role, it became natural for me to affirm it by offering a workshop entitled "Coping with Hearing Loss." The key word, "coping," indicated where I thought the emphasis belonged. I felt challenged by the notion that, instead of bewailing the neglect and indifference of society, I myself ought to assume the responsibility to help to effect change, even if but a little.

For weeks, wherever I moved about town, I carried pen and notepaper in my purse or my pocket. Even in the supermarket, I caught stray thoughts and scratched notes on my shopping lists as I moved my cart up and down the aisles. Watching a television program, I lost the thread of the story as some idea for a workshop intruded on my consciousness.

With a book on my lap, I would discover that I was about to turn a page without having absorbed a single line of print because I had been thinking about how to stimulate workshop participants to relax, how to overcome resistance to breaking the silence. I imagined different situations that might occur at the session and decided how I would deal with each one. My ears were sharply attuned to the words individuals used whenever they spoke to me about their impairment.

SEVEN

Workshops on Coping with Hearing Loss

Soon after we bought our home in Spartanburg, South Carolina, ten minutes by car from our daughter's house, we became involved in the community's Shepherd's Center, whose members are chiefly retired senior citizens. The center, a major attraction, reinforced our decision to move closer to Susan. The members are animated people who continue to enjoy life's abundance and opportunities. Some are former faculty members of the nearby colleges and religious institutions and are still involved in professional activities. Their scholarly contributions enrich the weekly programs. As program contributors they recruit faculty colleagues not yet retired and other individuals. Members in the audience get a taste of college or renew old experiences, perhaps with greater enjoyment than they had as students encumbered with term papers, grades, and exams. Weekly meetings provide the social environment for friends as well as cultural stimulation. They usually arrive early, exchange greetings, and rush to meet friends, to examine the day's program schedule, and to decide which sessions to attend.

In our second year of residence I acquired a strong preference for a front seat in the lecture rooms. By this time I had noticed that others hurried to reach the first and second rows. I saw that many of the men and women were using hearing aids but was not surprised to find that no one mentioned having a problem. Often when I introduced myself I explained why I needed a front seat, pointing to my hearing aid. I was rewarded by a warm expression on the faces of my neighbors—even those without any aids in their ears. I longed to talk about the problems that my impairment had caused me, and I hoped to learn from the experience of others. When I began to write on hearing loss for publication, I was further motivated to ask other people for their answers so that I could incorporate them in my articles. The popularity of the first two rows of seats reinforced my desire to carry out a resolve to help my readers understand and accept this kind of affliction. I then decided to take the next step by setting up a workshop at the Shepherd's Center.

I considered whether the fact that Lou and I were comparative newcomers would be a drawback. I felt encouraged by the southern hospitality we had enjoyed. Most of the members of the center appeared to be staunch natives of Spartanburg or other southern cities, proud of their heritage. Having lived most of our lives in New York, we had problems with the high-pitched southern drawl and with dialects that seemed to vary even from one area to another even when no great distance stood between them. It was not easy to recognize "hahr" as "higher" or "reem" for "room." People from some place in North Carolina tended to add syllables; thus the hem of a skirt became the "hee-em." I was initially mystified by "pinney," which proved to be "penny." I felt as if I were learning a foreign language, and because of my hearing loss, I covered my confusion with a forced smile. Sometimes, when people seemed to be asking me a question that I could not understand, I didn't know what to do and sensed impending disaster. This problem with dialects added to my concern that we might forever be known as "New York Yankees" to our new friends. I saw that I was daring to initiate a program for local residents who "belonged," as I did not. Like a tourist in a foreign land, I increased my knowledge of things that were associated with the South: the foliage (crepe myrtle and magnolia blossoms), the food (grits and hush puppies and the ubiquitous southern fried), fishing (catfish, bream, and bass). I studied the road signs commemorating historical places (Cowpens, Walnut Grove plantation).

Warm southern sociability made me more conscious of my stiffer Yankee reserve. I abandoned the hasty "Hi!" or "S'long." My daughter explained, "You don't rush a southerner. It isn't like meeting an acquaintance on an errand in New York City." I could no longer get by with a brief nod of recognition in the supermarket or simply walk toward my table in a restaurant. Instead, I soon realized I must allow plenty of unscheduled time to stop and participate in a leisurely conversation. When we stopped at a gas station and had to wait our turn, there was a long delay while the man who had just filled his tank chatted with the station attendant about a mutual friend.

Almost from the first introduction, I was deluged with gifts. When my doorbell rang, I often found myself greeted by someone carrying a token of goodwill to the newcomer: homemade bread, tomatoes from the garden, a bag of the famous South Carolina peaches or the precious Vidalia onions, even a whole salad arranged like a colorful mosaic on a big round platter. All this generosity taught me to respond accordingly. Alas, I found I was never able to catch up. Whenever I reciprocated with my honeyed stuffed cabbage or raisin-studded buttery biscuits, a suitable return was not long in coming. I needed time to understand and absorb the genuineness of "southern hospitality," which, I learned, lived up to its reputation. "They really mean it," I exclaimed to Susan, describing the bounty that elicited my admiration of the southern spirit. Nobody ever disparaged "Yankees" to me or said anything that might be derogatory about people "up north." That would have been a breach of courtesy that seemed to be instinctive.

Even as I enjoyed such warmth, I felt myself an outsider, for only two years had passed since I had come to live in the area. Would a New Yorker setting up a workshop in this community of the Deep South be viewed with suspicion for displaying northern aggressiveness? Had I moved too fast? Would people react by ignoring the program invitation? What if, when the day arrived, no one came?

To allay these misgivings I drew upon the memories of previous occasions when I had suffered similar fears following a burst of ambition the initiation of some new activity. I recalled the day I was offered a promotion at work; the day I started to teach my first class of forty adults at a university; the day I agreed to compose and deliver the opening devotional service at an important annual meeting of several hundred top-level staff of the National Council of YMCAs. I remembered that each time I had leaped a hurdle and achieved a new level of self-confidence and skill. Best of all, each time I had taken supreme pleasure in the experience apart from feeling gratified at having done something that others enjoyed. This time I did not divulge my present anxiety, even to Lou, my dearest friend. Such a confession might threaten the self-esteem I needed to carry the whole thing off. Instead, I concentrated on designing a well-organized, effective program and kept so busy that I had little time to dwell on my apprehensions.

As a new member of Self Help for Hard of Hearing People, I studied in each issue of the journal the short paragraphs that described successful programs conducted by the various local chapters. Most of these addressed two of my own major objectives: personal sharing of experiences and advocacy for nationwide concern and support. I believed then, and do now, that the deepest need of people with hearing loss is the courage to speak about their experience, from early warning signs, through denial, embarrassment, fright, and guilt, to the ultimate refuge of solitude. All the other pressing needs could be better dealt with after the release afforded by such therapeutic sharing.

Occasionally I came upon some reference to the biggest tragedy of Beethoven's life, a hearing loss which became the musician's secret burden from the time he was only twenty-eight and prompted a lifelong obsession with suicide. I was tantalized by the brief quotations of his words which I read in the musical notes while attending a concert. Because of my reverence for Beethoven's music, I wanted to know more about him. I scoured the library shelves. My curiosity was satisfied by Maynard Solomon's biography of the composer. Published in 1979, this book was rich with new information that the author had succeeded in extracting from letters and notations that had become accessible after centuries during which a long list of biographers had been at work, searching out and corroborating the facts. One entire section in the book is devoted to the musician's devastating impairment. I copied statements made by Beethoven himself, in 1801 and 1802, at age thirty-one and thirty-two. They described with striking familiarity exactly what I and countless others had endured more than a hundred years later. I planned to share these passages with workshop participants, for I anticipated that such material would break down resistance and encourage the exchange of personal experiences.

Below is a passage from a letter Beethoven wrote to his brother Carl which he intended for delivery after his death. In this document, which was found among his papers, he confessed that he was already beginning to contemplate suicide:

> From childhood on, my heart and soul have been full of the tender feeling of goodwill, and I was ever inclined to accomplish great things. But, think that for six years now I have

been hopelessly afflicted. . . . Though born with a fiery, active temperament, even susceptible to the diversions of society, I was soon compelled to face the prospect of a *lasting malady*. . . . I was soon compelled to withdraw myself, to live life alone. . . . It was impossible for me to say to people, "Speak louder, for I am deaf." Ah, how could I possibly admit an infirmity in the *one sense* which ought to be more perfect to me than to others. . . . for me there can be no relaxation with my fellow men. . . . no mutual exchange of ideas. I must live almost alone, like one who has been banished. . . . what a humiliation when someone standing next to me heard a flute in the distance and I heard nothing . . . a little more of that and *I would have ended my life*. . . . it was only my art that held me back. (Solomon 1979:116–17)

In 1801, too, he confessed in a letter to his dear friend Franz Wegeler:

For two years I have ceased to attend any social functions, just because it is impossible for me to say to people, "I am deaf". . . . And if my enemies, of whom I have a fair number, were to hear about it, what would they say. . . ? I have to place myself quite close to the orchestra in order to understand what the actor is saying, and at a distance I cannot hear the high notes of instruments or voices. . . . But if anyone shouts, I can't bear it. . . . I have often cursed my Creator and my existence. (Ibid., p. 113)

What a pity that Beethoven could not have had all the help that is available today. When I compare my fate to his and remember that my loss is offset by hearing aids, telephone amplifiers, television assistance, and a variety of other electronic gadgets with the promise of even greater inventions to come, all my anguish subsides.

I credit Self Help for Hard of Hearing People for much that I have learned. Contact with this organization helped to reduce my anxiety about my new project. The background literature plus a steady stream of new material that arrived

WORKSHOPS ON COPING WITH HEARING LOSS

with each issue of the SHHH journal assuaged my misgivings. No matter what happens to my hearing, there will continue to be improvements in technology to keep abreast of my increasing loss. I began to focus, rather, on the world outside. I wrote the organization about my dream of organizing a Spartanburg chapter. The staff at the main office promptly expressed enthusiasm and sent along a manual of instructions. Encouraged by their support I determined to revive my administrative and leadership skills, which had been dormant since my retirement. I had a responsibility to launch an experiment that would open up communication between hearing-impaired people and those with normal hearing in both South Carolina and Florida. The following notice appeared in a weekly bulletin distributed to members of the Shepherd's Center:

Spartanburg, South Carolina

Program notice—Meeting on October 9, 1986

Following the luncheon today Charlotte Himber will be conducting a special one-hour class on coping with hearing loss. This will be a one-time session. Mrs. Gayle Chaney, head of the Audiology Department at the South Carolina School for the Deaf and Blind, will attend this workshop to discuss the technical aspects of hearing impairment in the elderly and to answer any questions.

Mrs. Himber is a recent member and resident, originally from New York City, where she received an M.A. in Psychology at New York University. While working there toward a doctorate she was an instructor of courses in self-understanding and interpersonal relations. Besides her current published articles on hearing loss, her articles on family life and child development have appeared in national magazines, professional journals, and the *New York Times*. Her main bread-and-butter job was as editor of the national publication of the YMCAs of the United States, distributed to the professional staffs of the 2,000 YMCAs in the United States and in foreign lands. It focused on community programs geared to serve each age group and on overall family concerns.

I planned my introduction and typed a copy for use if it seemed appropriate. I knew that the circumstances might dictate a more spontaneous opening, but it was comforting to have something prepared in advance.

What is it like to be hearing impaired? Those who can hear well think they can tell, but those of you who don't know that they reveal by their reactions that they cannot. You have probably been subjected to their vain efforts to accommodate your loss. Instead of raising their voices just a little, they shout. If the talker is a loquacious person or excited, you are bombarded with sounds you don't understand. In a noisy room words generate a conglomeration of echoes. As they try to enunciate more clearly, they exaggerate their speech, so that your attention is drawn to their distorted features, while you watch for clues on lips, eyes, cheeks. They get tired of the exertion, yet you find it necessary to ask them to repeat. To relieve the strain, they tend to cut off conversation altogether, perhaps making some excuse to leave the scene. Thus ends the whole scenario.

I have thought often about how to describe to people who can hear normally how it feels when tones that reach my ears are diminished, entangled, uneven, when sound splits up from a faint rustle to a blast of thunder, then recedes as I try to rescue some meaning out of the confusion. I explain to them how each person's impairment is as unique as his fingerprints, especially in the case of presbycusis, the loss due to aging. There are a few general characteristics, however. In addition to the loudness, which often goes beyond the tolerance level, the words are distorted, so that while we hear them, we cannot understand them.

Because I have become so open in revealing that I am hard of hearing, many people seek advice, asking numerous questions about the loss they have been experiencing. Often it is a loss they have endured for years and not dared to admit—a common pattern I can understand only too well.

When my loss became so obvious that my family and friends acknowledged they knew of it, I found it almost impossible to describe to them exactly what happens while I am trying to listen.

Here is an exercise which I learned about in the course of much reading that is recommended by several practitioners. I suggest that you try it with your family, at home. Ask the individual to select a favorite program on the radio, and follow these instructions.

Tune the program to the point where it is most clear. Then shift the station dial slowly away from that spot, so that the words become foggy, rasping, garbled. At this point, turn the volume dial up slightly, and continue to listen. If the speaker uses numbers, you will be unable to distinguish "fifty" from "sixty"; you will hear the word "consist" and it may reach you as "insist" or merely "sit." Try it for fifteen minutes, keeping the dial at this point and stay with it as long as you can bear it. How does it feel? Now shift the dial back to the pure tone. . . . How does that feel?

Most likely your partner would give up long before the fifteen minutes, but even a few minutes is enough to increase understanding. This playful little simulation gives those who hear well a better idea about being hard of hearing. Not entirely, however! Think about all the changes in the environment that are encountered in a day in the life of a handicapped person. There is the telephone, the restaurant, the classroom or lecture hall, the theater, the traffic. Each situation raises its own unique kind of distortion and harassment. This experiment seems like a simple procedure; I can vouch that it is not! You will need to be very persuasive and patient, for your partner finds it too disagreeable to go beyond the first few minutes—even the first minute. But it pays off if it helps your relationships. Otherwise, even a slow decline in your hearing, which is most likely in the elderly, can be a serious deterrent to maintaining daily communication.

My plan was to ask Gayle Chaney, the audiologist, to proceed with a simplified presentation about the parts of the ear and how they function so that we not only hear sounds but also receive the message in the brain for comprehension.

The day of the workshop finally came. My knees were shaking when I entered the meeting room. I was startled to observe that I was followed by some thirty people. Many were in a hurry to get seats nearest the podium and settled down quickly. There was an air of excitement in the crowded room.

I had guessed right. The subject of the meeting had found an eager audience. I tested the microphone, helped by smiles and nods as people found themselves able to hear clearly. I introduced Mrs. Chaney, a young mother of two preschool-aged children. She came prepared with large charts and a supply of booklets and summary sheets to be distributed at the close of the session. Her voice was resonant and pleasant. She enunciated with professional clarity at a pace that did not exceed her listeners' capabilities. She placed several charts against the wall and called attention to the literature piled on the table nearby.

"You don't need to take notes," she said as several people groped in their bags for pencil and paper. "It's all in these booklets and sheets. I'll pass them around later."

Using her charts for illustration she described the anatomy of the ear and the two most common types of impairment, conductive and sensorineural, the latter being the one most often diagnosed in the elderly as presbycusis. She paused occasionally to allow her listeners to ask questions. I was happy to see that the audience paid close attention and asked highly specific questions which the speaker answered fully.

Now came a challenging part of my program design. It was suggested by the name of the organization Self Help for Hard of Hearing People. I described the origin of the word "educate," which is derived from the Latin *educo*, "to bring up, to lead forth." In this sense, the word "education" was formed to denote a process that teaches one how to draw from *one's own potential* the substance one learns to apply.

Through small group interaction, I anticipated that each participant would learn from the mutual sharing of personal experiences and acquired information. It was a method I had used successfully in my courses at the university on self-understanding and interpersonal relations.

I asked the participants to shift their chairs so that they were divided into subgroups of six persons. I explained that small group interaction would make it easier for them to communicate, whatever the level of their hearing loss. I distributed a sheet of questions that the groups could discuss with one another (see table 1). I suggested that those present with normal hearing distribute themselves so that there would be one or two of them in each small circle. The workshop groups would then more closely resemble average social gatherings of the same size.

Gayle Chaney was invaluable as a resource person. She busily responded to requests from individuals in the various groups and was able to confirm participants' statements, supplementing with some appropriate technical detail. Because I had studied the subject so thoroughly over the past several years, and because of my experience as a facilitator in the interpersonal communications process, I found that I, too, could function adequately as a resource. The room buzzed with excitement as each group became involved in sharing. I felt wonderfully alive as I hurried from group to group and saw how each participant experienced the relief of self-disclosure, how a flash of recognition crossed each face when a familiar story revealed a common experience in living with a hearing loss. Mrs. Chaney remained during this entire period of minisessions. I was able to deal with many of the social problems that participants want desperately to discuss because I had encountered the same sorts of stumbling blocks.

When the excitement subsided and I noticed a slowing down of energy, I announced we would reassemble as a

Table 1. Questions on Hearing Loss for Workshop Discussion

1. Talk to each other about your first awareness of a handicap. Tell how you finally decided to do something about it. Did you go to an audiologist?
2. Do you wear a hearing aid? If so, describe the period of adjustment to the aid. Ask the group to suggest ways of living with an aid.
3. How well do you do with television? the telephone? Share any suggestions you have.
4. Do you use any other assistive listening devices? If so, describe these and their value to you. What suggestions can you offer about the choice of device and how to make the best use of it?
5. Describe your communication with family and friends. What are the problems? What suggestions do you have for improving communication? Do you take responsibility for telling your listeners specifically how they can help you? Tell the group what works and what doesn't.
6. How candid are you in acknowledging your problem to store clerks, cab drivers, telephone operators, sales people, and others? What suggestions do you have about such encounters?
7. What developments would help you manage your impairment better?
8. Brainstorm about information and ideas you would like to share with the public as regards hearing impairment, treatment, training, and so forth.

total group. I called attention to a small pile of evaluation sheets on which people could anonymously comment on the session. The atmosphere in the room had undergone a significant change; casual acquaintances, or people who had not known each other at all, had become close and friendly in two short hours.

A recorder from each group reported the highlights of the minisessions. Each group seemed to have made one or more observations that had not been made in the other five groups. The variety reflected the diverse personalities and experiences and confirmed my belief that subgroups were worthwhile when the original group was large. I made a mental note to repeat the format whenever the circumstances warranted it.

Luckily, I had used my tape recorder as I moved among the small groups and during the recorders' reports. I now had a substantial list of the kinds of questions that people were likely to ask in such situations. Later I contacted Gayle on several occasions to check the validity of the answers that the participants made to the questions during the sessions. I kept careful records of the fine supplementary professional data she gave me. This material formed the basis for the question-and-answer sections in appendix 2 of this book.

The success of my first workshop confirmed me in my resolve to continue. When I read the enthusiastic comments on the evaluation sheets (which most of the writers had signed), I felt an exhilaration that banished all of my misgivings during the previous weeks. I was now more than ever ready for the next workshop, which I decided to hold in Florida, where we would soon be living during the winter months.

When we moved to our winter home in Port St. Lucie, I observed that many residents were wearing a hearing aid, although not one of them ever mentioned it in my presence. Sometimes I deliberately introduced the subject of hearing aids, to assess the response. There was usually some embarrassment and reluctance to continue. I hoped that by setting up a workshop in our retirement community I might break the silence.

Port St. Lucie, located halfway up on the eastern coast of the Florida peninsula, had been our choice as a winter residence because it was sparsely populated. Traffic was not yet the problem it had become further south; shopping was a breeze. We were lured by the lush southern foliage in the savannas, the variety of palm trees with their long, supple branches dipping and swirling in the breeze. Our friends up north, who had tried to keep us from "running off to the boondocks," teased us that we were surrendering prematurely to old age.

The environment has since changed. Port St. Lucie has been identified as one of the fastest growing areas in the United States, although those of us who have enjoyed it for a decade or more have not yet been troubled by the effects of growth. Fortunately, as population increases, so does employment, so that there is an influx of younger people and the community has a balanced mix of age groups. Conversing with youth, however, does tax the elderly, who are strained by the younger person's faster speech full of slick phrases, puzzling slang, and careless articulation. The time seemed ripe for providing hearing-impaired people with an opportunity to confront this challenge.

I provided the local weekly paper with a notice announcing a workshop entitled "Coping with Hearing Loss," which would be conducted at no charge for those who were hard of hearing as well as for those with normal hearing, especially people with hearing-impaired relatives. Again I suffered conflicting feelings. The community wasn't asking for my message. Why did I bother? Why couldn't I just enjoy the peaceful surroundings and allow the hearing-impaired elderly to keep their secret? I found I could not ignore my urge to voice so common a problem, to reduce some of the unhappiness I saw around me. I was sure that many people would be grateful for an end to the isolation induced by society's ignorance and indifference.

With the approach of fall I was reunited with my friends. Each year I noticed that more of them appeared to be losing their ability to hear and understand speech. I detected more hearing aids tucked skillfully under the thinning wisps of hair carefully curled over their ears, heard more frequently the familiar "What?" uttered with wrinkled brow and head cocked forward. Many spoke with raised voices, almost shouting. Still, would they consent to attend my meeting? I was surprised at how the attendance at various other meetings had declined. I scanned the folders laid out on the front desk of the clubhouse, where people signed their names to enroll in activities. Fewer and fewer of the older residents registered to attend Great Books discussions, lectures, and classes in painting, ceramics, wood carving, photography, and square and social dancing. Would "Coping with Hearing Loss" win out against the apathy of older residents who were finding it more difficult to stay involved and keep moving?

Each day I checked the sign-up folder for my program. Five names were written in after a whole week had gone by! Two days later, three more. I telephoned Michele Carpenter, the licensed audiologist who had volunteered to address the group. She had spent thirteen years as the clinical audiologist in a speech and hearing center in a hospital in Seattle and had supervised the audiology staff and services in one of the largest programs in the nation. At the present time she was director of the Hear Center in Port St. Lucie, which offered, in addition to the standard hearing services, counseling and community education through classes. I felt it was incumbent upon me to inform her that the initial response had been feeble. "Don't worry, Charlotte," she said in a cheery clipped voice that was resonant on my amplified telephone receiver. "I'll come and talk to them no matter how small the group may be."

My heart swelled with gratitude. Despite my fears, however, on the day of the meeting there were thirty-six names on the list! I checked the room for size and acoustics. Southern Florida was having a record cold spell, and we would need to use the heating unit. To my dismay, I discovered that its sound reverberated from the walls and the exercise equipment stacked against them. The heater made as much noise as a blasting machine. Elderly people are assailed by loud noise and distortion even when they have no noticeable loss. Such an invasion of sound would assault people with a serious hearing impairment like a rush of outside traffic. In this room there was no hope of conducting a workshop in which participants would contribute.

I chose a much smaller room and was helped in moving the chairs close together in the limited space. It had excellent acoustics and a newer, almost silent, heating unit. A few sturdy early arrivals lugged more chairs in from the large room. I knew that the thirty-six people would feel comfortably close for easy communication, and I even made room for two or three more. People who don't hear well feel a tension when they attend meetings with wide spaces of empty seats around them. Instinctively those of us who must constantly maneuver for the best transmission of sound have learned that people's voices are narrowly channeled and protected by close body contact in a crowd, so that vibrations aren't absorbed by empty spaces.

At the exact moment of the scheduled time for the workshop, to my surprise, the participants arrived en masse. For the first time I came face to face with the oldest people living in our retirement community. The group included many with whom I had lost contact because their infirmities had kept them confined to their homes. A number leaned heavily on canes, stepping forward hesitantly. Some were guided by spouses and friends with supporting arms. Several were shuffling forward carefully with the uneven gait of the arthritic sufferer, one leg bent, shoulders hunched, eyes riveted to the ground as they monitored each step. One man held up the line as he moved at a snail's pace. A woman just behind him informed me, using her lips without sound so that even he would not hear her, "He's blind too." He asked to be seated in the center of the first row, as close as possible to the speaker.

I was stunned into awareness of how the aging process can impose its brutal reality and thereby disrupt the serenity of retirement. But the scene changed promptly as the participants settled themselves comfortably, discarding canes, sweaters, bags, and other paraphernalia. The faces before me relaxed into smiles. I watched people greet each other energetically despite the feebleness of their limbs. They seemed happy to be there. The bright smiles reminded me that a person with a handicap may find it comforting to enter an environment in which everyone has a physical disability of some sort.

In my opening remarks I described my objectives: to provide a brief general description of the outer, middle, and inner parts of the ear; to invite discussion of the problems that we all experience; to encourage open and mutually helpful suggestions of ways to manage the problem; to elicit examples from one another who have improved their communication and, consequently, relationships with family and friends. We would learn about the various assistive listening instruments now becoming available in addition to hearing aids, some of which Mrs. Carpenter had brought along for demonstration. The smallness of the room precluded dividing the participants into subgroups.

I distributed several handouts during the session. One sheet outlined common hearing problems. One sheet listed specific suggestions addressed to normal hearing people, which participants could later share with their families and friends. I also included copies of one of the magazine articles I had written that described my own experiences in acquiring and adjusting to a hearing aid.

I introduced Michele Carpenter. Like Mrs. Chaney during my first workshop, she projected her voice sensitively, which helped her listeners to relax. She modulated her voice to an intensity appropriate to the confines of a small room and paced her sentences comfortably without exaggerating her words or articulating too precisely. Her eyes focused on the faces in the audience, and when she moved about she always continued to face them. She maintained the same level of sound to the very end of each sentence, so that the audience did not need to strain to catch her last words.

After a few casual remarks aimed at getting her listeners used to her voice, she began somewhat formally to speak. Almost at once hands shot up, demanding attention. She showed no displeasure at the interruptions; instead the questions were incorporated into her address and were answered in the order in which they were presented. The questions and answers lengthened her talk considerably. She obviously welcomed the interruptions as a means of enriching the content with material to satisfy the immediate need of each questioner, especially because all the questions dealt with situations commonly experienced. Eagerness to be heard, I should point out, is a characteristic of many hearing-impaired people. In fact, as previously noted, people respond to hearing loss in two diametrically opposed ways: by trying to sustain communication, which many achieve by doing most of the talking, or, conversely, by withdrawing to avoid the strain of a social situation. The audiologist was plainly delighted to see the audience become articulate so quickly.

The group of thirty-nine appeared to consist predominantly of talkers. I was not surprised. People's eagerness to speak showed that they felt at ease. Here any mistakes would be understood, and no one need feel inhibited by the possibility that something irrelevant would be said. Michele realized that her listeners desperately wanted answers to questions that had plagued them. Accordingly, she set aside most of her prepared talk and devoted the rest of the session instead to the many questions and shared discussions. She seized the opportunity to invite the participants to suggest ways in which people could help themselves. Her listeners responded with enthusiasm. Occasionally a person with normal hearing rose to contribute an idea. My husband drew a hearty laugh when he explained that he had learned not to try to get me to respond to remarks that he made "while the water was running."

Most of the participants had undergone a long period of initiation as a handicapped person, secretly harboring the shame of it and wary of being found out, of being labeled feeble, or senile, or just not very bright. Now they were exuberant, released from the cage of seclusion and misunderstanding. Under these circumstances, who would want to listen passively to a prepared talk and withhold questions for the end of the address? Like myself, they had long lists of concerns that they had withheld from their own families, subdued by the impatience they frequently encountered.

I taped the questions and answers on my recorder, as I had done in my first workshop in South Carolina. (These are also included in appendix 2). I noticed that although many of the questions related to the care and adjustment of hearing aids, some hinted at the joylessness of life for lonely old people with a physical loss, who yearned for understanding by spouses, children, or friends.

Bearing in mind the constraints on the energy that a hearing-impaired person can expend in a social situation, I watched for the first signs that the excitement was abating. When they came, I announced that the final item on the agenda would be a description of assistive listening devices currently available (see appendix 3). I reported that extensive research was underway, with the promise of further advances. When adjournment was announced, I asked the audience to complete the workshop evaluation sheets I had prepared. Almost everyone who filled out a report form used the word "excellent." Some stopped on the way out to thank Mrs. Carpenter and me. One woman stayed until all the others had left. She stood at the door and spoke in a shy, soft voice. "I know now that I'm not alone," she said, embarrassed by the tears in her eyes.

Later that evening I thought about the difference in the constituency of the two groups, the one in South Carolina and this one in a retirement community. The South Carolina participants were younger by an average of perhaps ten years. Their loss had not yet taken its toll in vigor and emotional energy. For the older people, the majority in the Florida group, hearing loss was one more infirmity to be endured in the late seventies and eighties. Worse, the adjustment to a hearing aid, always rocky, is more easily endured by those in their fifties and sixties. All the literature warns against delay in acquiring a hearing aid. It is easier for a younger person to get accustomed to the change in the sounds heard through an electronic device, to the sudden bursts of amplified intensity, distortion, and peripheral noises. Older people resist more stubbornly and often have periods when they utterly reject the aid. Those who came to the Florida workshop had had these experiences. They lacked the patience to listen to a lecture on the structure of the outer, middle, and inner ear or on the various kinds of hearing losses and diseases of the ear. In Spartanburg, this addition of educational material was welcomed as a reminder of student days.

My analysis of the two groups was to help me thereafter as I continued to develop workshops for coping with hearing loss and to meet with support groups that assembled informally.

EIGHT

New Skills and Future Prospects

This book has focused largely on the predicament that confronts the elderly after they reach sixty years of age. But we should not forget that the hearing-impaired population includes all age groups, from infants to seniors. The hearing impairment of one family member has an impact on the whole family, not to mention friends and other people with whom the afflicted individual communicates day after day. Everyone knows someone who is hard of hearing, and everyone is learning to make some accommodation, even in the most casual encounter.

As we look toward the future, technology will bring good news for everybody. Two of the most prestigious researchers and writers on audiology have said, "For centuries, the problem of how the hearing mechanism functions has been in dispute, and many books and articles have been written on the subject" (Newby and Popelka 1985:45). During the current decade more than in all previous years, however, scientists have made great progress toward understanding how we hear and toward creating the technology to correct the associated physiological failures. The pace of research today and the quest to perfect and apply the new knowledge promise continued improvement in the next decade. Moreover, the media and popular literature are proving more responsive to the problem, so that this "invisible handicap" is becoming less and less an affliction to be endured in secret. In the meantime, the hard of hearing can do much to help themselves.

Speechreading

Recently a picture flashed before my mind's eye of my employer in an office where I worked during the summer after my freshman year in college. It was my first office job, and I was scared. In the large organization I could not conquer a vague uneasiness about this man, who was the head of the accounting department. He was tall and elderly, lean and dapper, with a high forehead crowned by a healthy crop of shining gray hair. Whenever I met him, I was uncomfortably aware of his piercing gaze, which made me feel oddly guilty. A few days before I left to return to college, I noticed him consulting a telephone repair man who carried a supply of tools clipped to his belt. There was an air of conspiracy about their conference. One of the permanent employees who had helped me during those trying weeks whispered that, because the accountant was becoming increasingly hard of hearing, he had been urged to try a new kind of listening device suggested by the phone company that might help him keep his job as a department head.

After I became hard of hearing, the face of this troubled man loomed sharply in my memory, with that insistent stare which had intimidated me. In those days, being hard of hearing was a dread secret, far worse than it is today. Exposure might call into question one's competence as an employee. I realize now that this man had merely been trying to speechread my words because he couldn't hear them clearly. The method is loosely called lipreading, because the teaching has focused on the movement of the lips.

To understand the process, watch your features in the

mirror while you talk. Say the word "same." Then say the word "lame." The whole configuration of your face changes when you produce the *1* sound. Now repeat "same," and notice the half smile around the cheeks. "Lame" draws attention away from the cheeks, upward toward the lower lids of the eyes. A portrait artist sees this difference clearly and knows how to depict the distinction.

I have given a literal description of lipreading, a technique which concentrates on interpreting the minute changes caused by the movement of the lips. It is difficult for people who have grown up with normal hearing to learn. People who were born deaf or who have had a profound hearing loss for many years have had more practice in living with their handicap and have eventually learned to lipread with ease. Today, the term as it is applied to the hard of hearing more accurately refers to speechreading. It is taught at hearing centers and by speech pathologists who conduct lessons in formal classes.

Teachers of speechreading follow a broader curriculum. They train the student to make the most of residual sound capability by incorporating many visible clues to understanding. The expression in a speaker's eyes adds to the meaning of the spoken words; it can change the tenor of a question from challenge or hostility to sensitivity or concern. Meaning is conveyed by a variety of other spontaneous facial expressions and by the rise and fall of inflection, the changes in pitch to match the emotion behind the words. All the body gestures—even pauses—can be significant, as most stage humorists affirm. Instruction includes the skill of deducing the meaning of an entire sentence from a key phrase or word, the gist of a paragraph from a single phrase, or the overall message of a speech from the gestures of the speaker.

Actually everyone uses all of these strategies while listening. Studies have shown that the average listener may not "hear" more than 60 percent of the words spoken. A group of research psychologists investigating nonverbal messages concluded that feelings of liking or preference during communication are conveyed

- 55 percent by facial expression and eye contact
- 38 percent by the tone of voice that is used
- 7 percent by the words used.

In routine communication, apparently everyone uses powerful resources other than bare words. The hard of hearing are forced to rely more heavily on a variety of strategies some of which they eventually invent so that, even without special instruction, they keep building up their skills. These are acquired to some extent automatically while the users constantly improve their attentiveness. Such a process is not unusual; anyone who lives with a handicap acquires compensating mechanisms.

A professional speechreading therapist does not emphasize individual sounds or comprehension of one word at a time. Therapists sometimes start by demonstrating how much we are already accustomed to speechread. They may begin a conversation by speaking in a very low voice or using almost no sound at all and ask the kind of questions most of us hear frequently. For example, "What is your name?" "Where do you live?" "What is your phone number?"

The student will gain confidence from this experience, and the therapist will form some impression of overall readiness. The exercise makes a good beginning for a working relationship. The student learns that the objective is to acquire general understanding of what is being said, without expending time or energy on trying to catch each single word. The important thing is to keep pace with the speaker by grasping the meaning of whole sentences and even paragraphs whether or not some words are missed. This method of listening, in fact, is used to some extent by all speakers, but the hard-of-hearing person must learn to summarize more quickly and become resigned to accepting the inevitable gaps. A therapist is careful to refrain from the temptation to speak in a loud voice or with special attention to enunciation, as doing so will slow the development of skill in speechreading. It is better for the speaker even to exaggerate the low voice, almost to a whisper, to entice the listener to attend.

Since the ability to hear accurately when a speaker mentions clock time and calendar dates is vital, there is early training with numbers. The importance of understanding numbers can readily be appreciated. Hard-of-hearing people may experience many situations of inconvenience, or even real disaster, from failure to hear such details. There is therefore likely to be a session on numbers used in money or time, with words such as "one," "ten," "dime," "quarter," "ten dollars." Numbers "eight" and "nine" are easily confused, as are "fifteen" and "sixteen" and "fifty" and "sixty." Students are advised to ask for repetition during a conversation when numbers are involved, for example, by asking, "Did you say your address is eight twenty-five?" In schools or hearing centers such skills are usually taught to groups of people who have the same goal and reason for learning. A procedure involving mutual self-help and reinforcement develops. There is also the stimulus of good-natured competition and the group's mutual interest in the subject under consideration.

Not everyone needs to consider taking formal lessons in speechreading. Some good speechreaders have never had a lesson; for them the years of practice were sufficient. I have acquired most of my skill by reading books with chapters on speechreading and by following the procedures they describe. I read the material over many times, each time gaining a better understanding and ability to remember what I have read as I use the instructions in my normal encounters. (See the bibliography for recommended works on speech-reading.)

People who have no problem with their hearing cannot fully appreciate the stress involved in the daily effort to concentrate that must be exerted by a person with partial hearing. The pace of speech among young children, and especially among today's teenagers, is usually torturously rapid, and young people have great difficulty in slowing down for Grandma. Grandma, wanting desperately to maintain ties with her progeny, tries not to show that she is not understanding all that is being said lest her relatives decide to visit less often. This strategy of deception may frequently produce a laugh on both sides, but sometimes it results in abrupt silence and mutual bewilderment.

A great deal of energy is expended in speechreading, which requires the listener to watch for visual clues and apply any understanding of the background of the subject being discussed. This activity is taxing to the listener trying to keep pace with the words that continue to flow from the speaker. Something similar happens when a person who is just learning a foreign language is carrying on a conversation with a speaker in the speaker's native tongue. The dialogue usually ends sooner than it otherwise would; the listener wants time out to rest. For this reason and others, people who are hard of hearing crave solitude and tend to decline social invitations or space them far apart.

Auditory Training

Auditory training, another survival strategy, is training in using residual hearing most effectively. It entails learning to distinguish specific speech sounds, for example in words that are similar (examples are "near," "fear," and "dear"), and the voiceless consonants, such as s, f, p, t, sh, th, and so forth. Confusion of these sounds is common in neurosensory loss, which elderly people constantly complain about (even those who are unaware that they have begun to lose hearing acuity.)

The therapist focuses on the specific speech area in which the pupil has difficulty, as indicated on the audiometric tests for word discrimination. A properly prescribed hearing aid should take into account the speech frequencies that give the hearer the greatest difficulty in discrimination, but even the hearing aid cannot completely overcome the problem. Training should increase the discrimination score so that the message transmitted to the brain becomes intelligible. The value of a custom-designed auditory training program therefore depends on the accuracy of the hearing evaluation. It helps people who are exceptionally troubled by the amplification of sounds from a hearing aid.

"Turn your hearing aid up," my husband keeps urging when I ask his help in understanding the words in a television program.

"I *have* made it louder, as loud as I can stand it, but that only makes it worse."

Hard-of-hearing people are affected not only physically but emotionally, socially, educationally, and spiritually. Nevertheless, they should not retreat to a separate world. Speechreading and auditory training can be tremendous assets for the speaker and the listener and are well worth cultivating to the limit of one's individual capability. They are the key elements to staying in touch with one's social environment.

Preventive Care

You can protect your future by shepherding the hearing you now have. The hazard of loud noise is the price we pay for the sophistication of our industrial technology. According to researcher Edwin Rubel, who spoke at the 1987 annual meeting of the American Association for the Advancement of Science, brain cell damage from infancy on may markedly affect the ability of the brain to process sound signals and make them intelligible. Very loud and persistent noise is a major cause of such damage. He recommended that to protect their offspring, pregnant women should avoid exposure to continuous very loud noises. No one can escape the noise of traffic while walking down a city street—pavement construction machines, trucks grinding over potholes, shrieking sirens, and boom boxes. One audiologist showed me her custom-made earplugs. She carries them with her in her purse, to use while she waits on subway platforms or when she is merely out walking. Consider acquiring earplugs if you plan to attend sports events, protest meetings, or any event where the volume of noise may escalate. If you don't have custom-made earplugs, even a set of the ordinary commercial ones will be of some help. Use a shoulder bag to hold personal needs and small packages so that your hands will be free to cover your ears quickly with the palms if you are suddenly assaulted by noise.

Modern household equipment imposes daily trauma on the hair cells of the inner ear. The chief culprits are vacuum cleaners and garbage disposals. Dishwashers, laundry machines, cordless telephones that may be shrill when held close to the ears, and many other appliances emit noises that pound on your eardrums. Turn your hearing aids down or move to another room if you can. (Ask for help from a spouse or other family member.) Have your hearing and hearing aid checked regularly, at least once a year. The aid may require professional cleaning or other adjustments you are not aware of. Your audiogram may reflect changes that require a new hearing aid with a more modern mechanism.

Although you should resist the temptation to refrain from socializing, you will enjoy your friends more if you avoid meetings that trap you in a noisy situation. A busy restaurant poses a real threat to the hard of hearing; in fact, most of your guests will have just as frustrating a time there as you, although they won't usually admit it. Instead, they raise their voices to drown out the voices of diners at the next table—who promptly try to outshout them. On holidays, when restaurants are crowded, schedule your celebration a day ahead or a day later. You'll win kudos from the management and will probably enjoy much better service.

Where you sit in the restaurant becomes important. When you're about to be seated, or even beforehand, ask the person in your group who is taking charge to advise the hostess that one person in the party is hard of hearing. You don't want to be stuck near the kitchen, in a traffic lane, alongside a counter where a busboy empties trays of dirty dishes and silverware, or in the center of the dining area, surrounded by a circle of tables with diners jubilantly imbibing their third cocktail. The first time I asked one friend to make such arrangements for the four of us, she said she'd "feel funny," so I offered to do it myself. I was surprised to discover how easy it was, and I was also surprised by the kindly response of the hostess. When we came again to the restaurant, the hostess recognized me and led us to the table she had specially reserved when we phoned. Now this sort of request has become routine procedure for my family and friends.

Future Prospects

Research and experimentation centers on the construction of hearing aids take advantage of the latest advances in biotechnology and microprocessing. The scientists are concentrating on the number one problem with nerve deafness—the muffling that makes speech hard to understand, even with amplification.

There is continual improvement in lowering the interference from background noise, a problem that has plagued all users of hearing aids. When they amplify sound, they also amplify the oppressive, distracting background clamor. At the Gallaudet Research Institute and elsewhere, work is continuing on devices using computer technology to improve specific sound articulation. It is to be hoped that further refinement of the aid mechanism geared to each individual's area of loss in a specific frequency will be more successful in solving the problems of background noise. The mechanical aid will more precisely adjust to those sound frequencies at which correction is needed and will not amplify the sound where no amplification is required.

The tiny in-the-ear canal aid which was widely publicized when President Reagan was fitted with it has been hailed by thousands of new users. It is suitable for a mild to moderate loss. Many who have been unable to overcome their reluctance to be seen wearing an aid are grateful for this breakthrough. We can expect improvement in such miniaturized units, so that even people with greater loss will ultimately prefer them if they have retained enough manual dexterity to be able to insert them. Already one model of aid on the market is said to control the volume of sound, minute by minute, so that the elderly need not struggle to adjust the volume as the environment changes and the wearer moves about during the day. One company now offers a digital "microimpulse volume control," which may be operated simply by touching the hearing aid.

Behind-the-ear aids and devices worn on the chest—models which are both still necessary for some hearing-impaired people—are improving. To help individuals with a profound hearing loss, electrotactile devices applied to the skin are being developed which will produce sound waves that vibrate to alert the wearer. For people who have been deaf most of their lives, there are cochlear implants that transmit sounds electronically and, when the user is trained, can improve interpretation.

The Food and Drug Administration has now approved a bone-conduction mechanism hearing aid that is implanted in the skull. The unit is connected to a minimicrophone. This device accomplishes the effect that Beethoven discovered over a century ago when he pressed his forehead against the piano keys to allow the sound to penetrate the bones of his skull. People with middle ear damage will derive more benefit from this device than from the common hearing aid. Several weeks after the surgery, the patient dons an external unit which receives the amplified sound magnetically, bypassing the middle ear. Even tinnitus sufferers (about 20 percent of the people in the United States) can anticipate some relief. Patients can be fitted with more effective masking devices to drown out the annoyance of continuous buzzing, hissing, whistling, and other head noises. More accessible training in biofeedback and management of stress will help the patient who is emotionally exhausted from the constant onslaught of internal noise.

In the meantime, hearing loss has become an issue of national concern. Mark Medoff's play *Children of a Lesser God*, about a deaf girl, became a popular film. It was widely viewed throughout the country. Lou Ann Walker's book *A Loss for Words*, was a bestseller. Not long ago striking students protested the appointment at Gallaudet University of a new president with normal hearing. Thousands of television viewers around the nation tuned in for days to scenes showing Washington crowded by supporters of the Gallaudet students. They poured into the capital to add their voices to the protest. The students won their goal when the appointee resigned to enable the board to choose a successor, Irving King Jordan, Jr., a graduate of Gallaudet, formerly dean of Gallaudet's College of Arts and Sciences. The news appeared in headlines across front pages.

All over the United States, people have begun to listen to the hearing-impaired population. Thanks to the advocacy role of the American Association of Retired Persons, Self Help for Hard of Hearing People, the National Association for Hearing and Speech Action, Gallaudet University, the New York League for the Hard of Hearing, and numerous other national, state, and local groups, as well as various congressional representatives and senators, advocacy programs have intensified and are bringing results. At this writing, there are bills under consideration in both the House and the Senate to create assistive listening devices for the deaf and to make telecaption decoder programs more widely available. In the fall of 1988, the Senate and House Appropriations Committee agreed to spend $96.1 million to fund the National Institute on Deafness and other Communication Disorders.

Apart from their value in educating the general public, these activities are finally eroding the individual resistance to the acceptance of personal hearing impairment. We may look forward to the time when hearing loss will no longer be called "the invisible handicap," when hearing aids and new assistive listening devices will be used with as much freedom and dignity as eyeglasses.

My heart pounds with excitement at such signs of the public's awakening. Through the media I am able to redefine my identity: I too am a normal person. The bridge erected between the two worlds at last allows the hearing handicapped to cross with confidence and composure. And the breakthrough is being maintained; the media continue to carry personal stories and news relating to deaf and hearing-impaired people.

People who are hard of hearing are prone to withdraw from social participation. As they grow older, they often become accustomed to isolation. New developments, publicity, and technological advance will encourage them to stay in the mainstream and to remain in contact with others. Only by so doing can they continue to enjoy and contribute to the diversity of human life on this planet.

My best advice is: to learn to remain close to people; stay in the hearing world. Whether you are the speaker or the listener, you can bestow a gift of love by the depth of your attentiveness.

AFTERWORD

From my childhood I remember Tanta, my mother's older sister, now gone. Everyone in the family knew about Tanta's intuition. Her insights, which she impulsively shared with us, were accurate and needle-sharp. She had a genetic hearing impairment and often lapsed into long periods of silence to allow her ears to rest while the others at a family gathering continued to chatter away. In time she gave up trying to hear and instead used her eyes. She studied faces, the twist of a lip, and lines of laughter or distress. She noticed gestures, hands at elbows, and fumbling with skirt hems, belts, and buckles. She was alert to the subtleties in a phrase carelessly uttered and casually ignored by the rest of us. Her sudden astute remarks, often made after the general hubbub had died down, or sometimes even a day or two later, were for us a source of delight. She showed great tolerance of the human frailties that we displayed in our sometimes insensitive and acerbic family gossip. She seemed to find life entertaining and enjoyed watching the farce and drama that she could distill from the scraps of conversation that reached her eardrums. She lived quietly content, filled with kindness and patience despite her affliction. The lesson she taught was that as the sense of hearing diminishes, the other senses strengthen. Long after Tanta's verbal contributions faded, her wisdom continued to enrich our lives.

APPENDIX ONE

Coping with Hearing Loss: Some Practical Suggestions for Better Communication

Ten Commandments for People Who Live with a Hard-of-Hearing Person*

1. Be patient. Remember that a person who is beginning to suffer hearing loss is like a child beginning to talk, to listen, and to understand. All the conditions of communication are changing.
2. Accept reality. It changes both of your lives and introduces new elements in your relationship. It isn't going to go away. Reconcile yourself to the fact of your spouse's loss as you would to the loss of a child's arm. It doesn't change your spouse, the one you have learned to live with.
3. Speak slowly. Consider what it's like for you when you listen to a newscaster on television who rushes through lines, especially when statistics are being quoted.
4. Don't shout. It doesn't help, and it may give the impression that you're angry. Learn to speak distinctly. Careful enunciation is a useful habit to cultivate anyway.
5. You may recall the famous line in a Broadway play "You know I can't hear you when the water's running." Adapt it to include: while the television is on, when the

*My husband created these ten commandments. They reflect his experiences as the nonhearing-impaired spouse of a hearing-impaired person.

washing machine or the dishwasher is running, or when someone in the same room is carrying on an animated conversation on the telephone. People with hearing loss find it hard to block out sounds while they are straining to hear your words.

6. Don't talk with your back to people with a hearing loss. Even if they can't read your lips accurately when you face them, they will get a better sense of what you're saying.

7. Don't start walking away while you're still talking. Your words will come out as "I'm going to see if . . ." Frustrating, isn't it?

8. Agree on a signal that you can use in company when your hard-of-hearing spouse is talking too loudly. People with a hearing loss often cannot hear their own voices well enough to judge their loudness.

9. Don't show annoyance because you must repeat or because the hard-of-hearing person seems to have forgotten something said a few moments ago or even yesterday. He or she probably didn't hear you the first time.

10. Have a heart. Hearing loss is worse for the afflicted person than for anyone else. Consider that you may also have to learn to live with your own hearing loss someday. That's one of the prices we pay in this century for living beyond the biblical "three score and ten."

Tips for Effective Communication with Someone Who Is Hard of Hearing

1. Agree with me on a signal that can be used when: my voice is too loud; I'm monopolizing the conversation; my response is totally irrelevant because I heard wrong (clue me in as unobtrusively as you can, or simply repeat some key words of what was said); I've interrupted because I failed to notice the speaker hadn't finished. If

you can't catch my eye with your signal, try to tap me on the shoulder.

2. Keep hands away from your mouth while you're talking. Also avoid scarves, cigarettes, and gum. Either trim your mustache or raise your voice.

3. Face me when you talk to me. Otherwise I need to keep moving, following you to get the whole message. If you need to leave the room, wait until we're together again to continue.

4. Don't shout. It distorts the words. My hearing aid does the amplifying. But don't drop your voice as you reach the end of a sentence.

5. Most people speed up their speech when they get excited or in a hurry. It embarrasses me to ask you to slow down, so if I do it once, try to remember as you continue talking.

6. Don't exaggerate your enunciation. It makes you look different, and you are harder to understand. Sometimes you look funny, and I try not to laugh.

7. Don't call out from another room "I'm here." I may rush to get to you on the porch, when you're calling from the bedroom. Say "I'm in the bedroom."

8. If I've gotten a whole sentence wrong, if you will repeat *some* of the words the message that travels from my inner ear will reach my brain in time for me to catch up while you keep talking. It may even be better if you use a few different words to say the same thing, because the sounds you use the second time may be in a range that I can hear more easily.

9. You may expect me to hear as well on our porch as in the living room. But I usually hear better where there are soft drapes and carpets—anything that absorbs the peripheral sounds.

10. If you're having a lot of trouble communicating with me, I may have had a hard day and feel tired, or I may be

coming down with a cold or have a pain. Please make allowances.

11. When you talk to me on the phone, go slow, and re-phrase a few words if I don't catch on the first time. Don't raise your voice. Rely on my hearing aid to do the amplifying. I can adjust it if I need to, and I will get less distortion from it than I will if you shout.

12. Turn the light up in the room if it's dim so that I can "read" your face. Remember, too, that I can't read your face if there's a window right behind you or a bright lamp. At such times your face is a dark silhouette.

13. Whenever you want my attention, a touch will do better than words.

14. Use gestures and point to objects to clarify the meaning.

15. Don't just talk about dates, times, and places. Write them down.

16. Large groups in the room make it hard for me to follow the conversation, especially because someone is always interrupting the speaker or talking at the same time. You can help enormously just by repeating a few key words now and then. Do it privately, if you can.

17. If instead of saying "please get me a drink" you extend the sentence to "a drink of water," if I've missed the first part I will still know what you've asked for.

18. When you introduce me to someone, please try to artic-ulate well. It helps also when you add, "She's Cindy's math teacher," or "He's the father of your cardiologist." (Such an introduction helps people with normal hearing too. Try it!)

19. I know my loss must be a real burden to you. Please don't feel guilty when you've shown some impatience. I'm grateful for all you do to help me. I don't like it, however, when people show their impatience by signal-ling to each other as though I've said something silly or stupid. I can *see* even when I don't hear.

20. Come with me whenever I must see a doctor, especially the audiologist, because I am never sure I've heard these professional people correctly when they report a diagnosis and give me instructions.
21. During a lively conversation among friends in the room, when I've stopped participating, don't permit me to withdraw and isolate myself, even physically.
22. Tell me now and then how well I'm doing with my hearing problem. Exaggerate a little.

APPENDIX TWO

Frequently Asked Questions about Hearing Loss, with Answers

The questions that people ask who want to learn more about how to survive a hearing loss are endless. No single published book could cover them all because of the changes that are constantly occurring. This appendix draws on recordings I made during the workshops and during other group meetings, as well as on my numerous conversations with hearing-impaired people.

Living with a Hearing Loss

1. Q. Most of my friends are elderly, like myself. All of us miss some spoken words and ask each other to repeat. Are we all fated to suffer hearing loss?

   A. Not necessarily. Hearing impairment is described by audiologists as ranging from "mild" to "profound," but before reaching the first stage, "mild," people normally become less efficient in their hearing, and in other bodily functions, as a result of aging. We can't prevent some degree of loss. Even when a person is ten years old, some of the hair cells in the ear—there are about 30,000—wear out and die. Your ear does not replenish them. For a long time this deterioration largely affects the extremely high-frequency sounds, such as a piercing whistle, which technically measure 20,000 to 25,000 vibrations in cycles per second. Sounds at this frequency are much higher than speech sounds, which have a frequency rate of some 4000 to 8000 cycles, so that the deterioration does not become noticeable for a long time. The rate of deterioration, though inevitable, varies; with some people it is so slow and gradual that they never have a problem, while others may become hard of hearing in their forties or fifties.

2. Q. Now that I have grown used to a hearing aid, I function so comfortably that I feel that my hearing must have stabilized. How can I tell what is really happening?

A. Congratulations on learning how to live with a hearing loss! Everyone over sixty should be checked by an audiologist regularly, and those with a known loss should maintain a relationship with an audiologist who keeps a running record of the audiograms from year to year and can advise his client as to what is happening. Deterioration may be intermittent. You may find that a year or two passes with almost no change. As for permanent stabilization, it is not likely, but the deterioration is usually so slow that you can rely on a reserve of many years during which you will be able to function well, especially with the help of your aid. In the meantime, today's research technologists are diligently at work to invent new devices and improve existing ones; a competitive commercial market is monitoring their progress, so the millions of us with a hearing loss are justified in expecting to receive more help for the rest of our lives. All of us should be grateful that we live in an age when much is being accomplished to counteract the effects of our loss.

3. Q. A friend of mine who has a hearing loss reports that her hearing has been improving. It's true that she seems

to hear me better lately. Is it possible that her hearing has actually been improving as she is growing older?

A. Not unless the loss was originally due to an ear infection that has cleared up or to wax that had not been totally removed and has finally dried up and dropped out without her being aware of it. If your friend has continued to report such improvement over time after ruling out an infection or wax buildup, don't disillusion her! Thinking positively is very effective. In fact, she *is* hearing better because she has learned how to get the best results out of the residual hearing she possesses; you may have noticed that she has become very attentive when people speak to her. Also, she is probably positioning herself in a room so as to be closest to the source of sound. People with hearing loss often acquire these and other stratagems even subconsciously. They are remarkably satisfactory solutions to the common problems of the elderly. For example, I know that I automatically reach out to turn down the running water in my kitchen faucet when I am at the sink while someone is talking to me or when a television program comes on that I want to hear.

4. Q. Ads tell you that surgery sometimes helps. Is this true?

A. The most common type of hearing loss of the elderly is sensorineural (nerve deafness). This condition does not get better, and surgery won't help. Other types of loss, such as conductive hearing loss, may be treated medically or by surgery. Several types of diseases of the ear are treated medically. The otologist will identify these and administer treatment. For this reason it is essential for anyone who has trouble hearing to be checked by an otologist before an audiologist makes a prescription.

5. Q. My mother was invited to a seminar entitled "Coping with Hearing Loss" but refused to attend. She says she already knows very well how to cope. Is it fair for me to urge her to register for such a seminar if she doesn't feel the need?

A. This resistance is a natural reaction. People with any physical impairment usually want to downplay it in public. Tell her that *you* would like to attend the seminar because you want to understand her problems better. Your mother may welcome the opportunity to spend this time with you. You will both find that the group's sharing of problems is immensely satisfying and elicits many important suggestions from people who have devised solutions that work for them. People with normal hearing are as much in need of coping suggestions as their hearing-impaired living companions.

6. Q. As soon as I started using a hearing aid, my family expected all my hearing problems—and theirs—to be over. Their expectations don't match my experience, and I am still getting flack because I miss things they say to me. How do I overcome this problem?

A. Only *you* can explain to your family and friends that your aid has limitations. Tell them that sounds are different with a hearing aid, and your problems are not all solved. You still need their cooperation. Tell them you need to see their faces when they talk to you. Explain that talking to you from another room, or as you move around the room, or standing at the sink with their backs to you, makes it just as difficult to catch what they are saying as it was before. You will also need to remind them frequently not to raise their voices too loud and not to exaggerate their words, which causes facial distortion. Make copies of the ten commandments and tips in appendix 1 and distribute them to your family and friends.

7. Q.   I seem to hear better on some days than on others. Why? I may even remove my hearing aid on such days.

A.   On such days you may be at home, in relative quiet, with only one or two other people. There is also the factor of surrounding noises you don't control, like the sound of rain or a strong winter wind. I have found that the air pressure makes a difference in the penetration of sound. On a clear day when the atmosphere is sharp and the humidity very low, I hear better. When the humidity is high, sounds seem muffled—even people's voices rise as they unconsciously respond to the difference in sound penetration—and I have more difficulty distinguishing different speech sounds. There seems to be more distortion.

Temperature and light affect the behavior of sound waves. The relation of the sun to the earth at different times of the day may make it possible to hear at a greater or lesser distance, depending on the length that the sound waves travel within a given time as the earth circles the sun. These factors may account for some variations during a single day in your ability to hear.

On some days, too, you may not hear as well because you are tired or are coming down with a cold and are therefore less responsive to sensations, including sound. In this way you might perhaps recognize that you are due for a rest and should expect less from yourself.

Instead of discarding your hearing aid, keep wearing it so that you will adjust to atmospheric and physical conditions subconsciously, as people do who have normal hearing.

8. Q.   My work requires considerable airplane travel. I usually experience some discomfort a few hours after a long flight. There is a feeling of stuffiness, a slight reduc-

tion in hearing acuity, and occasionally even a little pain in one ear. Is there any danger of injury in my ear from flying?

A. Airplane travel poses some real concerns for anyone with hearing problems. You should pay a visit to an otologist if you have felt pain or actual discomfort in your ears from flying. You can minimize the danger by taking several precautions suggested by professionals. *Never* fly if you have a bad cold. Swelling occurs in the nose and may cause damage to the ear. In general, you can reduce the stuffiness, especially upon descent, by applying a decongestant to open the nasal passages and eustachian tube in the ear. You can purchase tablets or a nasal spray for this purpose over the counter. Use these about one hour before descent. Check first with your doctor, however, as they must not be used by people with heart conditions, asthma, prostate gland problems, high blood pressure, or drug allergy.

The above-mentioned considerations rule out flying for some people, at least at certain times. For most of us, there are several simple maneuvers. Chew gum or suck on a candy during descent and ascent. Yawn, swallow, or drink something while pinching the nose. If the stuffiness or discomfort continues for a day or longer, don't hesitate to consult a physician, who may need to treat you medically. It is advisable to wait before you fly again until you have felt comfortable for some time. For a more detailed explanation, write the New York League for the Hard of Hearing (see appendix 4).

The American Academy of Otolaryngology has published a pamphlet addressing the problems of hearing-impaired travelers. The pamphlet includes information on special amplification and visual alert devices, tips on how to make travel reservations, and additional sources of information. For a free copy, send a self-addressed stamped envelope to Travel Tips for Hearing Impaired People, American Academy of Otolaryngology (see appendix 4).

9. Q. Because I am severely hard of hearing I have not attempted to take even short trips by car if they require a stopover in a motel or hotel. Can you advise me how to manage such an experience?

A. Easy! Some hotels and motels offer a special service for hearing-impaired travelers. An example is the Hampton Inns chain. These hotels reserve a number of private rooms that carry a visual alert system to announce a fire alarm, a knock at the door, and telephone calls, all via a strobe light. They also have a telecommunications device for the deaf (TDD) reservation line so that, if you use a TDD, you can communicate with them visually through the typed message at both ends of the call. The TDD number is 1-800-451 HTDD.

An increasing number of other motels now set aside such specially equipped rooms. It's up to you to suggest that anyone helping you place a reservation inquire about this service. If everyone who is hard of hearing routinely asks for the service, such rooms will become increasingly available. The service should be free of charge. The president of Hampton Inns believes that since deaf and hard of hearing persons pay the same price as hearing people they should receive equal access to communication services.

10. Q. Since my husband became hard of hearing, we have been cutting down on more and more outings and invitations of the kinds we have both always enjoyed. His excuse is usually that he feels "too tired," and I readily comply with his request that we spend a quiet evening at home. Should I try, rather, to persuade him

to ignore his feeling of fatigue and continue to go out as we used to?

A. By all means. Of course you will need to gauge the extent to which his fatigue is a legitimate complaint. If it is not, and you indulge his request, you will only reinforce his subterfuge and interfere with the effort he should be making to use all the strategies discussed in this book that a hard-of-hearing person must learn in order to stay in the mainstream of society.

If you cater to his tendency to retire, you will help him develop a serious habit of isolation which will cause him—and you—far greater distress than the discomfort he must learn to endure if he is to continue to communicate with a hearing society.

11. Q. Why is there sometimes more distortion when I am using both aids? It helps considerably at such times to remove one of my aids.

A. Hearing loss is a very mixed bag. Some sounds in the words that are spoken to you you hear normally; others you hear only partially, with increased distortion when they are amplified. These differences may occur even within a single word. The hearing aid is not so magical an acoustic product that it will totally correct your hearing of a variety of sounds in a single multisyllabic word. (But the scientists are working at it!) If the overall distortion exceeds the benefit you are getting from the overall amplification, you apparently choose to go for less amplification by removing one aid. Try, instead, to turn the power down in both aids. In this way you will continue to have balanced hearing, which you cannot get from one aid if your loss is in both ears.

If your audiologist, as a result of your test evaluation, has advised you to stay with two aids, stick with binaural hearing unless you are in a modern building with excellent acoustics and the echoes are almost obliterated.

12. Q. A dealer tested my hearing and sold me a hearing aid. It works fine. Do I have to see an audiologist?

A. That may depend on the qualifications of the dealer. If, as a "hearing aid specialist," he has adequately completed the training that is now being recommended, you may have been properly fitted. Bear in mind, however, that an audiologist has had to undergo much more academic training to get a degree, and his examination will cover more than that of a dealer even if the latter is a hearing aid specialist. You will know for sure that you are using the best device available for your particular condition only if you have a thorough evaluation by an audiologist. At the present time most state laws stipulate that, unless you sign a waiver, no one may sell you an aid without your being examined by a physician (otologist) who can rule out the possibility of a medical problem. You may have signed the dealer's waiver at the time you visited him without being aware of its importance. The risk, in general, is up to you. You may decide to make do, considering the substantial financial outlay you made, but by all means see an audiologist for the recommended annual hearing examination when you are due for it next year.

13. Q. Why is it that, when I attend meetings in a large auditorium where the speaker uses a microphone, I often hear very poorly although the noise seems very loud?

A. How helpful a microphone may be in amplifying the sound usually depends on the placement of amplifying speakers and the acoustics in the room. In old buildings, a microphone is likely to raise the sound level of

the echoes as well as the original words. The reverberation time before the echo subsides may be one second or
as much as three seconds; in the meantime the speaker
continues to address his audience while the hard-of-
hearing person is still trying to sort out a past sentence
from the interfering echoes. Even people with normal
hearing are probably having difficulty. I find some improvement in these circumstances by moving around a
room before the program starts until I find a spot where
the echoes are less pervasive. Changing seats, of course,
is not always as easy to do unobtrusively if you wait
until the speaker is well into his address; your movement might cause considerable disturbance. Try to
gauge the problem from the first words that are being
tried out while the microphone is being tested or at least
during the opening remarks. People who use two hearing aids are usually at some advantage in dealing with
reverberation or conflicting noise. Generally, whether or
not the speaker is using a microphone, the size, shape,
and characteristics of a room influence how the voice is
heard. I personally have occasionally asked a speaker to
move his podium to a slightly different place on the
platform if it was originally placed too far to the right or
the left. Explain that if it is in the front of the room
everyone in the audience can face it without turning
right or left. Speakers are usually very pleased to follow
the suggestions of listeners, since such comments, after
all, indicate that the audience is eager to hear the
speech.

14. Q.   I have tinnitus, and the constant noises in my ear
bother me more than the fact that I'm hard of hearing.
Both the otologist and the audiologist told me there is no
cure for this or any chance that it will change. What can I
do to minimize the unpleasantness?

A.   It may sound cruel or insensitive for me to respond that you "learn to live with it," but most people with tinnitus report doing exactly that. Many have arrived at a personal solution; they turn on a radio very low to a musical program while they read or study or even during a conversation. Tinnitus can be masked by means of a device which most audiologists can provide that drowns out the noise in your ear. Background or environmental noise can also be an effective mask. Sears and other department stores sell masking devices.

15. Q.   We hear so much these days about the side effects of different medications. At seventy-three I need to rely on quite a few, and I have a moderate hearing loss. Are there any that may further damage my hearing?

A.   According to Singer and Brownell's (1984) research, reported in the journal, *Gerontologist*, you need to be alert to the following possibilities. Large doses of aspirin may reduce hearing temporarily; aspirin, if it is taken for long periods may even decrease it permanently. The same is true of antibiotics—streptomycin, neomycin, and so forth—and potentially of quinine, nicotine, and other drugs. Check with your doctors; they may need to consult the reports in the most recent journals to answer your question. Such a variety of antibiotic medications are available that it may be possible to change yours to safeguard your hearing.

16. Q.   My last hearing evaluation was done in a room that was not totally shielded from occasional outside noises. I could hear footsteps and even the faint ringing of the receptionist's telephone some distance down the hall. Wouldn't that interfere with the accuracy of the test results?

A. Most audiologists do not wish to eliminate peripheral sounds totally in the room where they do their evaluation. They get a more realistic report of your hearing in this kind of environment. After all, no one is likely to be in a scientifically soundproofed room at any time.

17. Q. Is there any indication that a specially designed diet may improve the quality of hearing? Also, I have heard some claims that acupuncture has a beneficial effect in alleviating hearing loss.

A. The relationship between diet and physiological deterioration involved in hearing loss among the elderly has received scant scientific support or investigation, although occasionally a researcher will cite some positive result from a study. An article by Marilyn Dickey in the *Washingtonian* (July 1988) states: "Anything that alters circulation can bring on some decline in hearing: high cholesterol, a high-salt diet, low thyroid function, nicotine, caffeine."

This subject is treated at length in Carmen (1983). Carmen emphasizes the importance of eating to maintain maximum health and resistance to illness, a program to which all of us should undeniably be committed. He provides examples of proper diet as well as information about the disastrous increase in chemical additives that *may* be contributing to tinnitus, hearing loss, dizziness, headaches, and so forth.

As to your question about acupuncture, Newby and Popelka (1985) write: "Some practitioners have claimed to 'cure' sensorineural hearing impairment through a series of acupuncture treatments. Unfortunately, otological and audiological studies of patients who have received these treatments fail to substantiate the practitioners' claims" (p. 96).

Learning to Use a Hearing Aid

1. Q. My mother finally succumbed to pressure from the family and consented to purchase a hearing aid, but she doesn't use it. Does her failure to use it mean that she has been improperly fitted or that she cannot be helped by a mechanical device?

   A. Not likely. Everyone has trouble initially getting used to a hearing aid. The process is not unlike getting used to eyeglasses the first time, especially if one is elderly. Show your sympathy and understanding of her reluctance and at the same time offer to stay with her as she tries to use the aid for a few minutes each day. Assure her that it is normal for her to resist it, and it's quite all right to allow herself as much time as she feels she needs—months, if necessary—but always gradually increasing the length of time, beginning with a quiet environment and one-to-one communication. Be careful to avoid encouraging her to practice with it in a situation where there is much background noise. If she likes to watch television, suggest that she do so when she's alone and there is no competition from the voices of people conversing in the same room. If time offers no improvement, schedule a visit to her audiologist to check the device itself. She may need an adjustment in power in the aid or some other change.

2. Q. Why does my own voice sound strange when I hear it while wearing my aid?

   A. This is a normal phenomenon and is not the fault of a hearing aid. If you have ever listened to your voice on a tape recording, you were probably surprised at how different it sounded to you. If the difference continues to bother you, by all means return to your audiologist or dealer and try different aids for comparison; if none seems to improve the sound, be assured that you will eventually get used to it and will no longer be concerned about it.

3. Q. My father appreciates his hearing aid but always asks someone who is close by to fit it in his ear because it keeps falling out. Once he dropped it on the floor; luckily it fell on a carpet, but now he's afraid to wear it, especially out of doors, for fear of losing it.

    A. It takes first users a fairly substantial period of time to learn how to insert the aid. This statement is especially true for an older person, who has probably lost some dexterity. The audiologist has undoubtedly reviewed the steps involved in mounting the aid in the ear, but the process must be repeated at home many times without the audiologist's support. If you rehearse the procedure with your father patiently, you will see an increase in his confidence that he has mastered the technique. Try this with him: have him stand in front of a mirror, holding the ear mold between his thumb and forefinger so that the canal portion is pointing into his ear. Let him gently push and twist until it fits snugly. He should not be afraid to press. The ear mold is as smooth as a baby's skin and can't hurt his ear.

4. Q. I've been using a hearing aid on and off for several months, but I find it very tiring. Everybody's voice is too loud, and I'm often embarrassed when I ask people to stop shouting and no one else seems to notice that they have been shouting. Is there something wrong with my hearing aid?

    A. Sounds you hear with an aid are bound to differ from sounds as you have been accustomed to hearing them naturally. You will tend to keep trying for a natural sound by increasing the volume. You have misjudged the amount of amplification you need to get the most efficient result. Try lowering it gradually; if you hear a whistling sound, the ear mold may not have been inserted correctly, and you are getting a louder sound than you need. Move the aid so that it settles properly in the ear opening, and the whistling will stop if you have turned the volume down sufficiently. Have someone talk to you standing three or four feet away in a regular voice, and adjust your aid until you can listen comfortably. For this trial, use a topic of conversation that is familiar to you. Now leave it alone, instead of trying to adjust it for each voice or each listening situation.

5. Q.   I was delighted when I first used my hearing aid in the audiologist's office. Now it seems to make me nervous and tense, and I have more trouble understanding conversation when I use it. I've practically discarded it. My family keeps pressing me to put it on; they don't believe me when I say I'm doing better without it.

A.   Chances are you have been trying to take too big a step in accustoming yourself to a hearing aid. Start all over. Use it for less than half an hour at a time and no more than an hour each day in your home when there are relatively few distracting peripheral sounds. Stay at this rate of use as long as necessary, until you can do so without feeling under a strain as you talk with anyone in your home. With some people the process may take only a few days; don't feel guilty or incompetent if in your case it takes longer. No one can say why the adjustment is different for some people. There may be some very subtle cause which science has not yet been able to determine. At any rate, it's not your fault! Simply plan on a program of self-indulgence, and allow yourself to extend this period of gradual adjustment in a relaxed mood. There are people who don't get there for a year or more! (I was one of these.) If you have the assurance that you have been properly fitted—you should possibly make another visit to your audiologist—you will finally make friends with this marvelous mechanical device.

6. Q. My hearing aid whistles when I press my palm against my ear. The noise can be very embarrassing when I'm with people and momentarily adjust my hairdo or tighten my earring. The worst time is when a friend greets me warmly with her arms around my neck and somehow brushes against my ear. The sudden whistle often produces a startled look on her face.

A. It may be that you are turning up the volume of sound too far. Test occasionally to see whether you can manage with a softer sound. If not, be aware that this kind of physical contact against your ear will usually cause some of that whistle. If you can't avoid the contact (who wouldn't want a spontaneous warm hug for a greeting?), the best solution is to explain at once, "That's my hearing aid. . . . See?" Then show the person that you are wearing one. Your friend will be grateful for your frankness, and you will be more comfortable and relaxed. It gets easier every time—take my word for it!

7. Q. As soon as I put on my aid I feel as though I have a tight plug in my ear. Is there anything I can do to relieve this sense of being clogged up?

A. The tight feeling is your assurance of a good fit. You will get used to it. A very light coating of petroleum jelly on the canal portion of the mold may make you more comfortable. Be very careful not to get any lubricant on the portion of the mold that allows the sound to penetrate. The discomfort should disappear in a few weeks. If it persists, the mold may be too deep or may otherwise not be right, and you will need to be refitted. You should consult your audiologist before making such a decision.

8. Q.   What can I do about the persistent irritation from a foreign body in my ear?

A.   Molds are made from two types of materials, one soft and one hard. The soft one is usually vinyl rubber. The hard one is acrylic plastic. You may be hyperallergenic to either type. If the irritation persists, you may need to change to a mold made from the other material. To do so you would need to see your audiologist. In the meantime, if the irritation has become so severe as to warrant medical attention, be sure to see a physician to prescribe treatment for the temporary solution. While a new mold is being made, keep the old mold. You may discover that the difference in the mold material does not solve the problem, in which case you simply need more time to get used to your aid. Also, even with a new mold there may be a need for several mechanical adjustments until you are satisfied that your aid is comfortable. While you are working on this problem, use your old mold as a spare. You can see from these explanations patience and conscientious efforts on your part and that of the audiologist may be needed to solve your problem.

9. Q.   There's an annoying itch when I wear my hearing aid. I have had my ear mold thoroughly checked. Since I am not otherwise allergic, my audiologist suggests that the itch will disappear as I get accustomed to using the hearing aid. Is there anything else I can do about the itch?

A.   See question 7 above about allergic reactions. Ask your otologist to check this. Otologists sometimes prescribe a liquid solution that you can apply lightly along the outer edge of your ear. They can also prescribe a different solution that can be placed right in the ear.

In my own experience, the occasional itch subsides in seconds and it works to simply ignore it. A persistent itch, however, can be very irritating. Your skin may become irritated from perspiration trapped in your ear; perspiration is salty and does tend to cause itching. To solve this problem I make a practice of washing out my ear opening with a soft sponge and lukewarm water (no soap) before retiring and sometimes even during the day. I then dry the area thoroughly, with a lint-free soft cloth followed by a slip of soft toilet tissue so that all the moisture is absorbed. Also be careful you rinse the soapy water out of your ears after shampooing your hair.

10. Q.   I feel very self-conscious about people noticing the aid in my ear; I often try to face people so that they see more of the side with the good ear. But every time I get a hair trim, my aid is relatively exposed for a few weeks. Can plastic molds be made to match individual skin tones?

A.   The skin tone in the opening where the aid lodges does not differ much from the surface skin tone. Moreover, your audiologist makes a selection from a variety of shades to match your skin tone. The problem more likely relates to your own awareness. Men's aids don't get much covering by most hair styles, but they hardly seem any more noticeable. People generally are not as interested as you imagine in peering at your ears, especially when they are paying attention to what you are saying. I change my hair style according to whatever costume I've chosen for that day. On occasions when I've told someone that I am wearing an aid for my hearing loss, the other person has often been surprised. Some people say, "I never noticed!" even though we've spoken many times before.

You will come to realize, as you read this book, that the best advice is to stop trying to hide the aid. If you are over sixty-five, you belong to the half of that population with a hearing loss. You can contribute to the progress of society in overcoming the resistance, as it was overcome in the case of defective eyesight. Fortunately this openness has become somewhat more common today, and you will be pleasantly surprised at how much easier it will become for you as you persist in working at it.

11. Q. My sister knows she is hard of hearing but says that as long as she can manage without an aid she'd rather not get one. Does this procrastination increase the rate of decline, or is it merely inconvenient to herself *and* to others when they communicate with her?

A. It certainly will not prevent whatever decline in hearing is naturally taking place, nor will it help her in any way. Actually the earlier she starts adjusting to an aid and learning how to use it effectively, the more likely she is to shorten the period of orientation. Besides, tell her that her family and friends will be grateful if she finally accepts the remarkable benefits of an aid, because this will also be helpful to them.

12. Q. My audiologist suggested that I ought to consider using two aids instead of just the one I've been wearing for the past year. I hesitate for several reasons. I don't like the fact that two aids would be twice as noticeable. Also, a second aid doubles the cost. I still find the task of putting an aid in my ear a chore, because I have lost considerable dexterity in my fingers. (Naturally, too, I can't help wondering whether the audiologist is influenced by the fact that he will profit from the sale.)

A. If you have a hearing loss in the second ear, especially if it is greater than "mild," the benefit from a second aid will be as great as the benefit from the first one. Furthermore, the sounds you will hear coming from both directions will be more balanced. I had to deal with this same question and will share my personal experience because it is typical. After I became accustomed to wearing two aids, I deeply appreciated my ability to hear and understand the sounds with less strain. I found I was missing less and was causing less annoyance to members of my family and good friends, the people with whom I communicated most. Music became stereophonic, and I enjoyed going to concerts. When you add up all of the benefits, you will not resent the additional imposition on your budget. Your relationship with your audiologist should be based on mutual trust. Most of these professional people don't make a recommendation on the basis of profit. I am assuming that you are both satisfied with the relationship.

What You Can Expect from Your Hearing Aid

1. Q.   How long should a hearing aid last?

    A.   On the average, about five years. Like other appliances, some aids continue to give satisfactory service longer. (One of those I use has lasted for nine years!) If it needs servicing after five years, have it repaired just once. If it breaks down again, replace it.

2. Q.   How much does repair cost?

    A.   The cost depends on what has to be done. A repair could cost anywhere from $45 to $135, depending on the defect.

3. Q.   When I wear my aid, all sounds get amplified. I have been warned to avoid loud noises, which may damage the ear. Is there some danger that the amplification from the hearing aid will cause further damage in hearing?

A.   In most cases of nerve deafness in the elderly, loss occurs in the range characterized as "mild," "moderate," or "moderately severe." The amplification from the hearing aid is not great enough to cause concern. The mechanism cuts off when sound exceeds the loudness which is safe. If the loss is "severe" or "profound," the aid needs to provide greater amplification, but the wearer will not be adversely affected because the loss is so much greater.

4. Q.   Occasionally I raise the volume of my hearing aid beyond even my own tolerance level. This happens while I am trying to hear something that is not clear, and I keep trying for a better result. Can I rely on my aid's cutoff point for protection?

A.   Yes. If the loud noise were to last eight hours without interruption, it would of course take its toll, but since you raise the volume only occasionally and turn it down again shortly, there is no danger.

5. Q.   I keep reading about a type of hearing aid which eliminates background noise. This is one of my greatest problems, but advertisers usually promise more than they can deliver. Can you tell me whether these hearing aids really live up to the advertising claims?

A.   A type of aid that cuts down background noise was introduced several years ago. The original model has been improved somewhat, but it still does not help everyone. The sensorineural loss of the elderly usually occurs in the high-frequency sounds. An aid that amplifies *both* the lower and the higher sounds proves a disadvantage for the lower sounds, which then become unnecessarily loud and more distorted. Your audiologist may be able to fit you with the newest custom-built model that aims to amplify only the sounds you are having trouble with, although so far users have not reported much improvement.

A digital system that is more sensitively designed may someday become popular. The sound is much clearer, because it eliminates the distortion in all previous models. It works so much better because it is not a miniaturized device of the sort now commonly used in the ear. There is ample room for the complicated technology that is used. It consists of three parts: a mold in the ear, connected by a wire to the aid behind the ear, and a processor worn in a pocket or attached to one's clothing. It is custom built in accord with the specific areas of hearing loss that the individual possesses. It is computerized to adjust continuously to the constant changes in sounds in a variety of frequencies as they occur.

It does have several disadvantages, and audiologists do not urge anyone whose loss is no greater than "moderate" or "moderately severe" to switch to it. As you would expect, it is very expensive—as of this writing it costs between $1,800 and $2,000 for a single aid—and two aids of this type must be worn. There are two other disadvantages. The processor is worn on the body and therefore calls attention to the impairment, and the processor is not an attractive object on one's clothing.

I find it comforting to know that such a distinctly improved system is available in case my hearing loss deteriorates from its present range of "moderate" to "severe" or even "profound." Now that we so often see people with normal hearing walking around with listening equipment attached to their clothes and receivers in their ears, I expect that hearing-impaired people will soon show less resistance to visible devices.

One more observation can be made about background noise. It is a fact of life in the current stage of noise-shattering technological sophistication. At least to some degree, people are used to it and have developed the habit of ignoring it, especially if they live and/or work in densely populated areas. A person with a hearing loss who begins to use a hearing aid is likely to be startled by it, not only because the aid amplifies sound beyond its usual intensity but also because sounds heard from a hearing aid differ somewhat from natural sound. The wearer must now learn to ignore peripheral sounds all over again.

There is no doubt that continuous loud noise is a threat to the organs of the ear. The Chesapeake and Potomac Telephone Company's *Visitor's Guide to Washington, D.C.* (Washington, D.C., 1987), includes the following bit of sinister humor: "A breed of deaf rabbits inhabit the area around the runways at Dulles International Airport. The noise of the planes is so great that in the hundreds of generations of rabbits since 1963, when the airport was built, deafness is their natural condition."

6. Q.   I have seen ads recently featuring hearing aids "in all the well-known models" that are remarkably reduced in price, some as low as $195. I have been paying about $600. What should a person make of such claims?

A.   Such low-priced aids are those offered to a person with a mild hearing loss, who may not even need to use a hearing aid at all. If you respond to this type of ad, be sure to read the fine print. Check to see whether there is a guarantee covering a thirty-day trial period during which you can return the aid at no cost except for the mold. If you respond to this ad by making a personal visit, you are likely to be told that in your particular case a more sensitive (and costlier) hearing aid is required. The retailer may use a hard sell to persuade you to buy other hearing devices of questionable usefulness. An audiologist told me that one of his clients had previously spent $1,000 on equipment he didn't need as a result of such an ad.

7. Q. Can a hearing aid cure your hearing impairment to any degree?

A. Nothing will replenish the dead hair cells in the cochlea of the ear, which caused the sensorineural loss. But because the aid increases your ability to remain in communication with the hearing society, you are less likely to isolate yourself. As you use your aid, you gain skill in speechreading and listening attentively. You acquire a variety of other skills that help you use your residual natural hearing to its maximum. For example, in any given environment you place yourself as near as possible to the voice; you choose your seat in a restaurant carefully. If one ear performs better than the other, you locate yourself in a way that gives you the benefit of your good ear, and so forth. Such constructive habits, which generally develop as you use your aid, do improve hearing to a considerable degree.

8. Q. Hearing aids are terribly costly. My audiologist told me that my aid should, according to the average, give me five or six years of service. That adds up to a considerable investment. Is there any chance that the price will go down?

A. I have been wearing one for nine years, and it is still in good condition. This is somewhat unusual, but other people have told me of similar experiences, so don't despair. In answer to your question, however, I am sorry to report that as the newer improved models come on the market the prices tend to go up rather than down, because the research that produced the advanced technology must be paid for. You will find that there is considerable variation in prices. A reliable audiologist will often even invite you to shop around, as mine has done. If you live in an area where there is competition among dealers, you may be the beneficiary and pay less. Dealers must charge enough to survive. Their prices are geared to the volume, the cost of doing business in that particular area, and their standards of service. As with anything else that consumers must have, you must evaluate a higher price against advantages such as convenience of location, reputation of the dealer, quality of service, and so forth before you decide what you are willing to pay. If your own audiologist sells the aid that seems most efficient for you, you should feel able to trust him or her implicitly to provide the many additional services you will receive during the first weeks, sometimes months, while you wear your new aid. Unless the difference is very substantial between the audiologist's price and that of a competitive dealer, you will probably choose to pay the former (as I have done).

9. Q.   There has been so much promotion of the tiny "canal aid" since Reagan began to use it that I am tempted to change to this model. Will it help me as much as the original in-the-ear aid, which I now use?

A.   If your loss is no greater than the middle range within the "moderate" category, it will probably be satisfactory. As of this writing, the canal aid has the drawback of being too small to contain the new automatic signal-processing technique that to a limited degree filters out unwanted or background noise. A larger unit is a better device in sound transmission and quality for the total range of hearing loss beyond the "moderate"; in fact, if people were willing to use a model even larger, such as the system that includes a processor to be worn on the clothing, they would find it superior. If you can overcome your resistance to wearing a device that is visible, you will not feel pressured by a dealer to change to a small model.

10. Q. A friend tells me she frequently finds her hearing has deteriorated and all she needs to do is see a physician, who removes the wax in her ears. I usually have my ears professionally cleaned only once each year and have never noticed any change in my hearing as a result. Should I have this done more often?

A. Your friend is lucky. Some people are persuaded to buy a hearing aid without first seeing a physician when they notice a loss. There are wax-producing glands in the ear which protect the drum membrane from dirt and insects. In many people the glands produce too much wax (cerumen), with the result that the excess must be removed more often to prevent the canal from becoming blocked. Only a physician should remove wax because the skin lining of the canal is very thin and sensitive and can be scratched. A bobby pin or other object may not only scratch the skin but may also cause an infection. By probing too deeply you can puncture the eardrum in addition. Your audiologist can check your ears and tell you whether to have a physician remove the wax more often than during the annual checkup. Apparently your ears do not accumulate excess wax, so you are getting the maximum benefit from the method you are using.

11. Q. When I first got my hearing aid, it fit snugly in my ear, and I had no trouble inserting it correctly after the first trial period. Now I find it much more difficult to insert. It doesn't go easily under the upper flap of my ear. I always feel I'm about to lose it; in fact several times I caught it in my hand just as I was about to adjust the volume. What is causing this trouble?

A. There are several reasons why an ear mold may no longer make a tight seal in the ear canal. You should have your audiologist check it. The ear canal itself goes through changes just like any other part of your body over the years. If the fleshy circumference has thinned out, the mold will feel loose. Even the movements of your jaw when you chew or speak may change the opening gradually. Sometimes the first sign that the mold no longer fits is frequent whistling feedback. This may be a signal that you need to have a new mold to seal in the sound and prevent leakage. A mold that fits well *feels right*, so that you find it easy to know when you have mounted it correctly; you'll feel more secure and will probably hear better. The cost will be only for changing the mold, not the aid itself, unless other changes have occurred in your hearing or in the aid proper.

How to Care for Your Aid

1. Q. How do I clean my hearing aid? When I bought it, it came with a rounded wire-tipped plastic stick about two inches long, and I was told to use it to remove any wax that I could see around the vent. I rarely see any, but what if a quantity of wax actually gets packed down into the vent where the wire cannot reach it?

   A. The wire-tipped appliance which was included in the sale of the in-the-ear aid at one time is no longer recommended because in probing the vent you might damage the mechanism itself. Instead the purchaser is given a soft brush which polishes the surface of the mold. You can safely rub it over the open vent. If you are still using the wire, discard it and ask the person who sold you your aid for one of these special brushes. If you cannot obtain one, purchase a very soft child's toothbrush; always be careful not to force the bristles down into the vent. If the mold has become sticky and needs more than this kind of brushing, use a dry, soft, lint-free cloth. *Never use anything wet*, as any moisture—even the humid air in the bathroom during a shower, can damage the aid. If the aid still seems sticky, audiologists can sometimes clean the surface with a buffing wheel. An aid should have an annual checkup in any case, during which the audiologist will if necessary clean the parts that you can't reach.

Molds that are attached to the behind-the-ear type of aid can be completely submerged in warm, soapy water, since all the hearing aid mechanism is in the unit behind the ear. If there is wax clogging this type of mold, it can sometimes be removed with a wire-tipped cleaner. An ear mold blower is also available from any local hearing aid dealer to blow out any wax. Before you clean this type of mold, be sure you know how to separate it from the hearing aid. Your audiologist or dealer will show you how to do this. Be careful at all times not to allow any water to soak into the hearing aid unit.

Still another cleaning method is used for the hearing aid in the frame of eyeglasses. The opening that leads to the microphone has a tiny hole that may clog. Don't try to clean the hole yourself, as you may damage the microphone. A hearing aid dealer can do it.

2. Q.   I dropped my aid as I was taking it out of my ear. Fortunately it landed on the bath mat. What may happen if I drop it on the harder surface?

A.   Don't! Make a practice of removing it as you incline your head over a table top, preferably over a table mat, but don't panic if it slips out of your hand. It has happened to me several times. I was at home, and it dropped once on a vinyl floor and once on a carpeted floor. Each time the battery still registered that healthy whistle when I turned it up high. What a relief! Most important: before you step out into the paved street, check to make sure your hearing aid is securely in place.

3. Q. I wear a tight shower cap when I shower. I have been keeping my aid on and have not had any trouble, as I use a very tight cap. Can I damage my aid?

A. You sure can! You've been lucky so far. The moisture in a bathroom, especially when hot water is steaming out of the faucets is bad for an aid. See that your aid remains dry at all times. If you tend to perspire, try to dry out the ear canal. Take the aid out occasionally on a warm day and wipe your ear with a soft, lint-free cloth.

An interesting new device has recently reached the market, the Dri-Doc Moisture protector. It is a water-resistant vinyl case to protect hearing aids from moisture. It is especially helpful when you need to remove your aid temporarily, for example at the beach, at poolside, in a locker room, or on the tennis court. Write to HARC Mercantile, Ltd., P.O. Box 3055, Kalamazoo, Michigan 49003-3055, or phone 1-800-445-9968.

4. Q. I have trouble with profuse perspiration. At times I can feel the perspiration running down my face and even in my ears. Is there any way to prevent damage to my aid from this moisture?

A. You have lots of company with this problem. First of all, don't attempt to dry your aid by placing it near heat or in the sun. Remove it when you use a hair dryer. You can purchase a "dri-aid" kit for only a few dollars. Ask your dispenser if he can provide it or a similar type of dehumidifier. On a warm day when you feel your body growing moist, remove the aid as often as you can conveniently do so, and thoroughly dry the ear canal. Always use a lint-free soft cloth for this purpose.

5. Q. I am continually hearing strange noises coming from my hearing aid. Is this a normal condition that exists in all aids?

A. I have checked with the advice given by Joshua M. Gendel, director of technical services at the New York League for the Hard of Hearing (personal communication, November 1988). He has described the various conditions under which such noise is to be expected and when it is a sign that your aid needs attention. I quote his complete response:

The first thing to do is to determine the exact type of noise. What you may be hearing is the ordinary noise in any environment, which is now amplified by the aid. Sometimes there is a defective component in the aid which generates a noise, and you cannot tell the difference. Find a quiet place and just listen. If the noise is no longer there, then you have been hearing the normal environment sounds—street noises, an air conditioner, a refrigerator hum. If the noise is still there and is loud enough to be annoying, you will need to get the aid serviced. You have to allow for some noise—like static—which some people may be more sensitive to, depending on the type of hearing loss even in a quiet place. This noise should never be so loud that it interferes with the sound you need to hear.

A type of noise that people are frequently asking about is the whistling, or feedback. This can be due to the aid itself or from a mold which has been fitted improperly. Press your fingers against the mold if you have this problem. If the feedback goes away and returns when the pressure is released, then your mold is the cause and you need to get it taken care of. If you have constant feedback, again you need to have your aid checked. A possibility with behind-the-ear aids worn by people who also wear eyeglasses is that the aid may tap against the glass frame every time a step is taken. Gluing a soft piece of material such as cotton on the aid or eyeglass frame at the point of contact can eliminate this problem.

If your aid has a telephone switch you may hear a hum when using it. This is normal. In these cases you need to make sure that you are not near an electrical device that is in operation, like a TV, a fluorescent light, or any electric motor.

6. Q. My hearing aid is insured for two years. What will it cost to repair it after that period?

A. There is no pat answer. If your audiologist can fix it locally, the cost will probably be minimal. If it needs to be sent back to the manufacturer, the minimum charge for checking and reconditioning it may be as much as eighty dollars. After that, it's a matter of luck! Wait for an estimate before you give your approval for the repair. If your aid is only two or three years old, it will probably pay you to have it repaired. If you have been using it for five years, consider you've had sufficient use to warrant the expense; go for a newer model incorporating recent technological improvements. Your new aid will probably give you more satisfaction than a repaired older model.

7. Q. Can I take out an insurance policy for my aid against theft, fire, and so forth?

A. People are not likely to steal an aid, although they may go for the pretty little velvet box in which you may be carrying it, thinking it contains jewelry, but there is certainly the possibility of loss, fire, accidental damage. The Midwest Hearing Industries as of this writing issues a policy that covers almost forty different makes of hearing aid, almost certainly including the one you are using, and the cost is very low, considering how expensive a new aid would be. This company will insure you against financial loss caused by theft, fire, accidental breakage, water, auto accident, and even what they refer to as "mysterious disappearance." They may repair your aid after "accidental damage" at no cost. The ad-

216

dress is 10 West Seventy-seventh Street, Suite 201, Minneapolis, Minnesota, telephone (612) 835-5232.

Questions about Batteries

1. Q.   How long should batteries last?

   A.   Battery life differs according to the number of hours the battery is in use and the length of time it has been on a store's shelf. Some of the batteries now come with a sticker on the mechanism that prevents deterioration while the battery remains in its package before exposure and insertion in the mold. If you choose to use this newer type, be prepared to pay more for it, but it's worth it. Variation in cost may in large part reflect battery life. The period in question may be anywhere from 25 hours to more than 100 hours, depending not only on quality but also (and principally) on the amount of use by the wearer. Ask about battery life when you make your purchase if there is no information in the literature with the package. You should shop around for the best price, as the battery for your particular model is standardized and clearly identified. The pharmacy of the American Association for Retired Persons sells these in quantities at a competitive price. If you are a member (you may join if you are over fifty), send for the catalog of pharmaceutical products and do your comparison shopping locally. The address for the catalog is: AARP Pharmacy Service, 6500 Thirty-fourth Street North, P.O. Box 14417, St. Petersburg, Florida 33733.

2. Q.   The battery for my old hearing aid used to last much longer than it does with this new aid. I seem to be changing to a fresh battery much more often.

   A.   Your new aid may have been made with more power because the audiologist believes you now require a stronger unit. There is considerable variation in the length of usage, depending on the power of the aid. You may be using your aid more consistently (which is good!), and the cost for additional use is well worth it.

3. Q. My battery went dead. I inserted a fresh one, and that didn't work either. I tried a third one, with the same result. I thought my hearing aid had conked out. It was very distressing because I had finally become very dependent on it. About half an hour later I tried again. All three batteries came alive and the aid functioned! What happened?

A. You may have had a tiny speck of dust caught in the opening where the battery is inserted. As you continued to work at it, opening and shutting the lever that closes over the battery aperture, the particle was swept away. The same thing may happen again. When it does, merely repeat the opening and closing process without the battery a few times. In any case, keep your aid in a dust-free place. The box in which it came when you purchased it is fine if you keep it clean and dust free.

4. Q. My battery went dead one morning when I inserted it, although it had been working perfectly all evening before I removed it as I prepared to go to bed. I dashed off to a hearing aid dealer, fearful that something serious had happened to my aid. He rubbed the battery on a piece of suede, and it was restored to life. Since he found no problem I felt foolish, but I wonder what really happened.

A. Your battery may have accumulated the slightest bit of moisture during the night when it was exposed, especially in the humid climate of Florida where you say you live. Keep your batteries in a cool, dry place at all times. When you remove it at night, put it into the (dry) box with your aid. Both belong in this box at all times when they are not in use. Rubbing the battery gently with the suede cloth dried off any dampness that had accumulated. (Also see question 3 under "How to Care for Your Aid.")

5. Q. I plan to do a good deal of traveling during my vacation in Europe. Will I have trouble getting batteries?

A. Probably not, but why risk it? Batteries come in a neat small container well sealed under plastic and may be packed with all the other small items in your luggage. The plane flight will not affect them if they are protected by the original unopened package.

6. Q. Can one get a type of battery that is self-charging, or a battery charger made especially for hearing aid batteries?

A. Not yet, but hang in there! All sorts of new devices are being studied by the hearing aid industry. Batteries aren't very expensive, however, if you purchase them in quantity and insist on the ones that display the individual stay-fresh stickers.

7. Q. My hearing aid has an on and off switch. Occasionally I turn it to "off," sometimes to reduce the noise around me, for example, that of a lawn mower or a garbage truck. These sounds are much louder for me when I wear my hearing aid. Also, at times when I'm alone I find it relaxing to cut out *all* sounds for a few hours. I do this by turning the switch to "off." Does this save wear on the use of the battery and make it last longer?

A. The battery will not operate or will operate only minimally when you use your "off" switch. Saving of the battery won't amount to much, however; don't be tempted to cut it off just for economy's sake. Bear in mind that some danger is involved. You may miss an emergency phone call, or other warning signals. If you're out taking a leisurely walk, you may not hear the oncoming traffic behind you. Instead of turning it off completely, merely turn it down to give you a sense of quiet, but allow enough sound to penetrate for safety, and forget about saving a few cents on the cost of a battery.

8. Q. Does a battery stop working all at once, or does it function at a decreasing rate of efficiency and wear out gradually during use? If the latter, would it be better to discard the battery before it has worn down completely?

A. Two types of batteries are most commonly used. Mercury batteries are readily available in many stores, even those which do not specialize in equipment for hearing-impaired people. They decline in sound quality when they are close to the end of their lives. You'd do well to discard them at this stage. Zinc-air batteries have now become popular. They last longer and consequently cost more but are worth it, especially because the battery is covered by a seal that should not be removed until you are ready to insert the battery in your aid. The seal keeps it from wearing out on the store shelf or in your bureau drawer. Usually you will be aware of no decrease in the sound quality until the battery is completely dead. Recently, however, I noticed that for a day or two before mine went dead there was a slight quiver in the whistle tone when I turned the volume up high. I learned from someone with a severe-to-profound loss that the voltage in her mercury batteries was more satisfactory *for her*. No single answer holds for everyone. You should discuss this subject with your audiologist.

9. Q.   Where should I store my supply of batteries?

A.   Pick a cool, dry place. Don't resort to the refrigerator unless you live in an extremely hot climate and do not have an air conditioner. If you must use the refrigerator, wipe the batteries when you remove them and hold them at room temperature for about an hour, during which time keep drying them as they accumulate moisture from the change in temperature.

10. Q.   Recently I purchased a "fresh" set of batteries and find that they are lasting for only a few hours. What's wrong?

A.   Either the batteries you purchased had deteriorated on the shelf, or they were defective to begin with. If a second set of batteries of a similar type purchased from a different source is giving you the same result, however, see your dealer or audiologist; you may need to have your aid adjusted.

APPENDIX THREE

Assistive Devices

The first effective assistive device is your own skill in listening, which you can acquire by ardent and patient practice. It took me some time to realize how much my own innate ability could help me.

First, I had to learn to pay attention, as all children are constantly being admonished to do in school. The older we get, the more we are likely to respond to distractions, because over the years we have amassed a vast store of experiences the details of which may suddenly be recalled by any of many stimuli. The brain's memory may be triggered by almost anything connected with what is presently happening. For a fraction of a second we are likely to stop paying attention.

Consider that you carry within yourself at all times this assistive listening mechanism: you can *pay attention*. Check yourself when someone else is talking to you and your thoughts have wandered. The speed of thought far exceeds the speed of human speech. On average a speaker may use four or five words per second, but the listener may be thinking three times as fast. What is happening during the additional brain activity? Unless you listen closely—pay attention—any extraneous thought will distract from the speaker. If you are using the time to concentrate on what is being said rather than on whether you turned off the light on the range at home or on how soon you need to leave to catch your commuter train, you are making the most of your listening skill.

Thus attentiveness, concentration, and avoidance of distracting thoughts and of peripheral noises all form part of your built-in assistive listening device. A few tips may help you. Ask your family and friends to attract your attention before speaking to you. At meetings, or in church or synagogue, avoid sitting near a door, a traffic lane, an air conditioner, or an open window, all of which will interfere with your concentration. Learn to feel confident in the way you're dressed, in your hair style and your makeup, and to ignore the bandage on your finger. These distractions may cause you to miss the very meat of a conversation. While nothing will keep you from missing some words—even normal hearing people miss some—by concentrating you will develop skill in grasping the content of speech.

Mechanical Devices

People generally regard a hearing aid as the only solution for the hearing impaired. Numerous advertisements describe other instruments which help bring the person with a hearing impairment closer to the normal hearing world. Some relevant information is readily available in audiologists' offices and in literature on tables in physicians' waiting rooms, but the general public has no curiosity about it. Even people who have been using hearing aids for years haven't taken the opportunity to learn how much additional help they can get at relatively little cost.

As I continued to write, research, speak, and conduct workshops, I too failed to take seriously the information in printed brochures that flooded my mail daily, at first because

I had learned to resist the hard sell that usually accompanied the ads. Besides, the wording was either too technical or was deliberately mystifying and complicated. Like all hearing aid users I had become skeptical of rosy promises. We have all had to learn from personal experience that our hearing aids fall short of some of the extravagant claims made for them.

Audiologists invited to my workshops began to bring one or two assistive units with them when I finally became interested and asked about them. To demonstrate how they work, they came laden with the necessary equipment, including their own televisions and yards and yards of wiring. Listeners in the audience took turns trying the devices. All of us were now ready to believe that we would be rescued from the fate we had feared—that the presbycusis of our advancing years might eventually defy all our efforts to keep abreast with life in the normal world. Below is a brief description of the major devices now available, all of which will continue to improve as a result of the current technological research. For the latest information, contact the organizations listed in appendix 4 and especially Self Help for Hard of Hearing People.

Several of the new devices, as I have noted, offer relief from the two main problems of people who are hard of hearing, namely background noise and distances between the speaker and the listener of more than three feet. Reduction in communication in these cases is minimized. It is not essential to turn up the volume because the speaker's words are transmitted directly to the listener's ears. Since amplification ordinarily increases the interference from background noise, the resulting distortion and muffled sound can now be controlled. Reception is relatively natural and pleasant. The benefit of all these mechanical aids is equally evident to people with normal hearing, whose patience is less strained during interaction.

Assistive Listening Devices

The Induction Loop   The loop, designed for use in small public rooms, classrooms, churches, and conference rooms, is suitable for people who have hearing aids equipped with a T coil. Listeners without an aid, or people who use one without a T coil, can purchase or rent a special receiver. The loop uses a wire or cable long enough to circle the perimeter of the room in which the audience is assembled. The wire is attached to the speaker of an amplifier, which is hooked up to the microphone. By means of a T coil, or the special receiver, the listener hears the speaker clearly without background noise. The loop can be permanent, installed on the floor or ceiling, or portable.

The FM System   As many as one in thirteen people in the general population have difficulty understanding a speaker in large auditoriums even where there is a good amplification system. Those who must use hearing aids will still have difficulty because their aids increase the volume of background noise as well as the sounds they want to hear. Nevertheless, in such circumstances hearing-impaired people do better with hearing aids than without them. Hearing-impaired people often choose to stay away from stressful environments such as theaters, large lecture halls, or worship services in large auditoriums. Without such cultural and religious activities, however, they feel deprived.

Assistive listening systems, the product of modern technology, are the answer. They work because they bypass the interfering effect of open space between the source of sound (as on a speaker's platform) and the listener. The hard-of-hearing person who is especially sensitive to the transmission of sound can now receive it directly in the ear. The intervening sounds have been blocked out during the process of transmission. Hard-of-hearing people can distinguish sounds they could not possibly receive otherwise, such as consonants and high-pitched sounds. This technology is so successful that even people who are not hard of hearing use headphones in large auditoriums or in theaters to make listening more comfortable. The FM system is one solution for this problem and others.

The FM system is an amplification system which facilitates communication for hearing-impaired people in any situation in which the speaker is more than three feet from the hearing-impaired person or in which there is background noise. It consists of a speaker-worn microphone and transmitter and a listener-worn receiver. The speaker's microphone transmits sound to the listener's receiver on an FM radio wave. Through one of several different types of receiver attachments the listener will receive the sound directly in the ear. FM systems have no wires or cords that attach the speaker's microphone to the listener's receiver. They thus increase the allowable distance between speaker and listener and thereby ease the communication situation. Because they are wireless, both speaker and listener can remain as much as 100 feet or more apart.

FM units can be used in any environment in which the primary speaker must compete with distance and noise in order to be heard, for example in auditoriums and other meeting rooms or in a car. The system works well because the speaker's voice remains within a few inches of the microphone at all times, so that the signal goes directly to the listener's hearing aid, effectively bypassing all surrounding noise.

Adults find an FM system beneficial in many situations. In the college classroom the instructor may mount a microphone on his clothing; the same benefits accrue wherever a single person is speaking or where one person speaks at a time.

I remember my surprise and joy when I was scheduled to speak to a school class of hearing-impaired children and found another type of FM system in use. When the supervisor came forward to introduce me, she deftly attached what looked like a little box on my belt. Then I noticed that the children were also wearing a unit of roughly the same size somewhere on their clothing. I found that I adjusted easily to the device and soon forgot all about it as I talked with the children. I moved around a good deal in the course of my presentation, amusing the children with gestures, and was not hampered by the box. I generally involve my listeners by asking questions. These children heard well enough to be able to respond appropriately.

FM systems have been found useful in board meetings, at dinner parties (for example in restaurants), in cars and buses, and in other noisy settings in which the hearing-impaired person is often left out. Use in these settings may require some adaptation on the part of both the speaker and the listener, but the benefits are well worth the effort.

The big stumbling block, as I can testify, is the hard-of-hearing person's uneasiness about exposure of the handicap, a feeling which precedes acceptance of the situation. Moreover, since women usually dress for parties and other festive occasions, they may hesitate to attach a unit to their clothing if it interferes with their costume. For me, the device is most easily used at a restaurant table when I am with people I know well who have become accustomed to my hearing difficulty. To fulfill my writing commitments I have found it invaluable in conducting an interview, once I have overcome my own diffidence enough to ask the interviewee's permission to use the system. I find it helpful to bear in mind that in the past, when I first started using a tape recorder for interviews, the interviewee would be self-conscious and somewhat tense. The awkwardness soon passed, however, as we both became interested in our conversation. I look forward to the time, still to come (and it will!) when the FM system will be as widely used as the familiar tape recorder and will cause no embarrassment on either side.

The Infrared System   The infrared device brightens my day when I spend hours watching television for news, information, and entertainment. It is appreciated by my husband too and by anyone else who is listening at the same time, because I can adjust the volume for myself without changing it for other listeners.

The infrared is a wireless system that converts sound signals into infrared waves, invisible light beams. The transmitter is plugged into a wall socket with a wire long enough to reach almost any distance in a fairly large room. The microphone is fastened to the front of the television speaker with Velcro (I have discarded the Velcro and let the little unit hang against the speaker for easy removal, because I often carry the device to a television in another room.) I use the cordless headset without my hearing aids. It is a very lightweight, flexible unit that hangs from my ears to below my chin and contains the volume control. I am not troubled by background noises, and the exceptionally clear reception reminds me of how the television used to sound to me before my hearing deteriorated. Best of all, I sometimes move about the room wearing the receiver with only a slight reduction in the quality of the television reception. During the hour while I am in my kitchen preparing dinner—a time when my favorite news programs come on the air—I can make the salad, stir the pots on the range, or tend the microwave without missing the "MacNeil-Lehrer News Hour," a favorite in our home. I do have to take some precautions; I will hear a buzz if I turn on a fluorescent light that shines directly over my head on one of the kitchen counters and when I turn my back on the sound source (for example when I lean forward to reach into the refrigerator). The receiver has a control that I can turn off completely at such moments. Most of the time I simply manipulate the volume as I move about.

My audiologist told me about a recently developed infrared system which costs less than $100. It has the advantage of allowing you to turn your back on the television, keep moving about the room, and still get good reception. When I tried this unit in the audiologist's office I was immensely pleased with it, as it gave me more freedom to move about. In my own home, however, I was not quite sure the reception from this system equaled in clarity that of the very much more expensive device. Perhaps the fault lay with my television or with whatever peripheral sounds were present in my large living room-dining room area. Because infrared systems are extremely sensitive, they amplify even the interference from the rustle of a blouse against the chest of the person wearing them.

None of the infrared systems can be used outdoors. (Mine once started to buzz suddenly when, seated near the television, I raised a window blind so that the setting sun shone brilliantly across my face. The bright sunlight interfered with the reception.) A second person can also use it, with an additional receiver. The same transmitter can be plugged into a socket in the room where a radio is being used. Those people who need greater amplification can purchase a different cordless headset to be used with a T coil hearing aid.

One of the many advantages of the infrared is that the personal receiver you use at home is compatible with infrared auditorium systems. You can bring along your receiver to use in theaters or large meeting places instead of using the receivers that are rented to the audience.

I paid $350 for the excellent model I chose after trying several less expensive ones, but it was worth it; I would feel very deprived without it. I hope that readers of this book will be able to purchase a satisfactory unit for less than I had to pay when the device was first put on the market.

Telecommunication Devices

Telephone Amplifiers   The telephone is both a friend and a foe to the hard of hearing. Dozens of times in a single day I find it an enemy that I must be prepared to confront. Fortunately, a number of weapons are available. I have personally used several.

First, I purchased a simple portable telephone amplifier from a local shop that stocks electronic equipment. A strap slips it over the telephone receiver, so that it is easily removed when the conversation is finished. It enables the listener to raise the volume of incoming sound. That system seemed to work fine in the store, and it is used by several friends who are delighted with the low cost. It gave me little help at home, however, whether I used it with or without my hearing aid, and the store clerk refunded my money when I returned it. Next I tried a unit that was lent me by an audiologist. This consists of a small device that is plugged into the telephone and rests on the table close by, where it can be manipulated by the user. This, too, gave me little help, although others have told me they find it sufficient; it is also a very low-cost item, and my audiologist took it back without charging me. You may wish to try both of these before going to the telephone company for the one I now use with great satisfaction. I purchased a new telephone from my local AT&T store that has a built-in amplifier handset that the listener can adjust during use and readjust for normal listening after hanging up. (Hold onto your original telephone as a ''spare'' if the new one should need to be repaired.) Your local store dealer may let you purchase the telephone on trial; you may return it and receive a full refund if you find it unsatisfactory. Everyone I know with this type of amplifier finds it extremely helpful.

There are many other adapters for the telephone. If you need help in locating a store that provides any of these, contact the AT&T Special Needs Center, 1-800-233-1222, or write AT&T at 2001 Route 46, Parsippany, New Jersey 07054.

A cordless telephone receiver that can be used throughout your home has been a boon for all those who cannot rely on the amplification in their own hearing aids when they use the telephone. I was unable to find one in any of the stores I visited that was satisfactory, although I tried many models. Radio Shack, however, as of this writing, has recently made available a cordless telephone that is amplified and compatible with hearing aids. This is particularly helpful to people with severe or profound loss. Ask for this model (the model number as of this writing is ET-425 Duophone, 43-553), and arrange for a trial period in your home. You may need to search for it in several stores. (By the time this book is published, department stores may have similar cordless telephone receiver models manufactured by other firms.)

Telecommunication Devices for the Deaf   The most popular device for the severely or profoundly hearing impaired is the TDD (telecommunications device for the deaf). It may sit permanently on a desk or may be portable. The portable models can be extremely useful if you are traveling and are not able to manage telephone conversations with the person who is most concerned about you. Both parties must have TDDs in order for a conversation to take place.

This unit will display a typed message on a screen that is attached to the receiver's TDD. If you are the one who is hard of hearing, this person will type out the message for you to receive on *your* unit. Some TDDs produce a paper printout—a permanent record of the conversation. Some telephone companies will rent you a TDD, for example, if you are traveling and want to feel safely connected with the person who is closest to you. The unit is very simple to use and assures that a message is never misunderstood. Although I am not severely impaired, I have considered purchasing one because there are times when Susan has some very specific information that I am unable to understand, and Lou is not always around to pick up the phone for me.

For more information (there are a variety of models and prices) contact the National Technical Institute for the Deaf in Rochester, New York. See the address in appendix 4.

An excellent pamphlet that describes TDDs and tells you more about any common problems in using them is published by Telecommunications for the Deaf, 814 Thayer Avenue, Silver Spring, Maryland 20910, telephone (301) 589-3006.

The Telecaption Decoder Anyone with a hearing loss, even if it is mild, often tires of the effort to understand speech on television, especially because the listening time sometimes lasts as much as one or two hours. At such times the telecaption decoder is an excellent substitute for hearing aids, especially if, like most elderly people, you "hear sounds but can't understand all the words." A printed narrative runs across the bottom of the screen and is broadcast at the same time as the program. It is visible only when a special "caption decoder" is attached to the television set. Even the spoken words seem clearer when the listener follows the printout. Usually any other viewer who is present and has normal hearing enjoys the additional help of a decoder, particularly when the broadcast features people who are not native speakers of English.

Many national network news programs are "closed captioned." Your television program guide identifies such programs with a small "cc" at the end of the program listing or the mark ⊊. The number of closed caption programs has been increasing steadily, thanks largely to the prodding of agencies such as the National Self Help for Hard of Hearing People and local chapter memberships, which have sent letters to the National Captioning Institute. You can join the crusade by writing to the NCI at the address given in appendix 4. At this writing SHHH has reported a "quantum leap" in captioned television programs, which include all of ABC's prime time shows and two-thirds of NBC's programs. PBS has increased its captioned programs, and CBS is beginning to do so. The AARP has been providing closed captioning of its televised programs for senior citizens. You can boost the effort by joining. AARP membership, which is very reasonable, has many advantages, including a subscription to the journal *Modern Maturity* and a pamphlet called *Have You Heard?* which is a remarkably clear and concise description of hearing loss with helpful suggestions.

Helpful video tapes are now also available, including one on speechreading strategies and one on sign language. A 1987 catalog provides details of loans, rentals, and sales. For a free catalog write National Technical Institute for the Deaf, Rochester Institute of Technology (see appendix 4).

In June 1988, the National Captioning Institute introduced its newest decoder, the TeleCaption 3000, with wireless remote connections to television, VCR, cable system, and satellite receiver. Ask for it in your local stores, or contact NCI 1-800-533-WORD for a listing of retailers near you that carry Caption 3000.

You may also be able to experience personally the pleasure of TV viewing by contacting a hearing center if there is one in your area. Hearing centers carry a variety of assistive listening devices for use with their clients.

Signaling and Alerting Devices

For people whose hearing loss is severe or profound, there are numerous alarm devices that use lights or create vibrations. You can purchase doorbell signalers, fire-smoke alarms, phone alert signalers, and wake-up alarms. Check your local department stores. For other sources, write to Nationwide Flashing Systems (see appendix 4).

The Hearing Dog

Hearing Dogs are an assistive device. They can help not only deaf people but anyone who has a hearing loss that is more than mild, from 55 decibels up, who usually uses hearing aids but removes them to rest or during sleep. Such people are in danger when they sleep if there is no one in the household who will hear sounds that might otherwise be missed but are important. The most satisfactory partnership results when you have your own dog trained. The animal is already familiar with the environment and owner and pet make a loving, trusting couple accustomed to accommodating to each other's wishes and needs.

The initial training is first supervised by a staff person in the Hearing Dog Program. This individual visits the home, "interviews" the dog and the owner, and examines the environment. Are there steps? Do carpet runners slip and slide? Is the door handle one which a dog can manipulate? Where are hearing aids kept while the owner is resting? Each home presents its own problems that need to be taken into account.

The dog will alert the owner to doorbells or knocks, telephone calls, alarm clocks, a baby's cry, or unusual sounds, such as those made by an intruder. Once alerted, the dog prods the owner and leads the way to the source of the sound.

For people who don't already own a dog, the organization contacted will provide one, usually obtained from the Humane Society; they will place it in a foster home for initial obedience training before bringing it to the new owner's home. Owners are also taught to train their pets.

You will recognize a Hearing Dog by its bright orange collar and leash. You will help educate the public if you tell people when you see a Hearing Dog because few people know about these animals. In forty-six states at present the Hearing Dog has the same legal rights as a Seeing Eye Dog. Hearing Dogs may enter restaurants, shopping centers, places of entertainment, and other public places. They travel with their owners on trains, planes, and buses.

Hearing Dogs behave like very will trained children on these excursions; they lie down patiently and scarcely move, waiting only for a signal from their owners that their attention is required. Often people cannot resist patting them. If you know anyone who has always been afraid of dogs it can be good therapy to arrange for that person to meet a Hearing Dog while it is resting beside its owner in a public place.

The program has been especially effective, because of the enthusiasm of the staff of the project, in South Carolina. The organization to contact there is the Southeastern Assistance Dogs, in the Speech, Hearing, and Learning Center, 811 Pendleton St. , 9-11 Medical Court, Greenville, South Carolina 29601. This group has been extending its services and has been publicizing such assistance even beyond the state. Its staff will advise you if you live in the Southeast. National program headquarters are the Hearing Dog Program, American Humane Association, 9725 East Hampden Avenue, Department HD, Denver, Colorado 80231; you may also write the Red Acre Farm Hearing Dog Center, Box 278, 109 Red Acre Road, Stowe, Massachusetts 01775. Many charitable associations cover the costs of placing and training Hearing Dogs, although if you can you are expected to help meet the cost. The program is comparatively new, and the number of such dogs available in your area may be limited.

APPENDIX FOUR

Resources

Alexander Graham Bell Association for the Deaf, 3417 Volta Place N.W., Washington, DC 20007 (Nonprofit; membership for children and adults)

American Academy of Otolaryngology, 1101 Vermont Avenue, N.W., Suite 302, Washington, DC 20005

American Association for Retired Persons, 1909 K Street, N.W., Washington, DC 20049 (Nonprofit; low-cost membership for people aged fifty and over; benefits include subscription to *Modern Maturity*, low-cost insurance, and inexpensive pharmaceutical products)

American Speech-Language-Hearing Association, 10801 Rockville Pike, Rockville, MD 20852, telephone (301) 897-5700

American Telephone and Telegraph Special Needs Center, telephone 1-800-233-1222

American Tinnitus Association, P.O. Box 5, Portland, OR 97207

Better Hearing Institute, 1430 K Street, N.W., Suite 600, Washington, DC 20005, telephone 1-800-424-8576 (Nonprofit; provides list of hearing care professionals in your area)

Food and Drug Administration, 8757 Georgia Avenue, Silver Spring, MD 20910 (Agency of the U.S. government; provides publications about hearing and hearing aids)

Hearing Industries Association, 1800 M Street, N.W., Washington, DC 20036 (Provides literature on companies that make or distribute hearing aids)

House Ear Institute, 256 South Lake Street, Los Angeles, CA 90057, telephone (213) 483-4431 (Communication assistance devices and information about them)

National Association for Hearing and Speech Action, 10801 Rockville Pike, Rockville, MD 20852, telephone 1-800-638-8255 (An advocacy organization; also furnishes literature and makes referrals)

National Captioning Institute, 5203 Leesburg Pike, Fifteenth Floor, Falls Church, VA 22041, telephone 1-800-533-WORD

National Hearing Aid Society, 20361 Middle Belt Road, Livonia, MI 48142, telephone (313) 478-2610 (An association of certified instrument specialists; to request a consumer education kit call 1-800-521-5247; for information on the National Board of Certification in Hearing Instrument Sciences, call [313] 478-5712)

National Hearing Association, 1010 Jorie Boulevard, Suite 308, Oak Brook, IL 60521 (Literature for public hearing care specialists)

National Information Center on Deafness, Information and Research, Gallaudet University, 800 Florida Avenue, N.E., Washington, DC 20002, telephone (202) 651-5051

National Technical Institute for the Deaf, Division of Public Affairs, Department C, One Lomb Memorial Drive, P.O. Box 9887, Rochester, NY 14623-0887, telephone (716) 475-6400 (Request current edition of ''Captioned Educational Videotapes'')

Nationwide Flashing Signal Systems, 8120 Fenton Street, Silver Spring, MD 20910, telephone (301) 589-6671 (Mail order and walk-in sales; product line includes signals for doorbell, telephone, babies' cries, alarm clocks, smoke detectors, decoders, etc.)

New York League for the Hard of Hearing, 71 West Twenty-third Street, New York, NY 10010-4162, telephone (212) 741-7650 (Complete services and instrument devices for people with hearing impairments from mild to profound; publishes bulletins on a variety of subjects for hearing-impaired people and their families; send for order form listing titles and cost)

Self Help for Hard of Hearing People, Inc., 7800 Wisconsin Avenue, Bethesda, MD 20814, telephone (301) 657-2248 (Membership organization; local chapters nationwide; bi-monthly journal, pamphlets, and extensive literature)

BIBLIOGRAPHY

An asterisk (*) indicates publications focused on speech-reading.

American Association of Retired Persons. 1984. *Have You Heard? Hearing Loss and Aging*. Washington, DC: AARP. (Free to AARP members)

Brackett, Diane, and Jane R. Madell. 1983. *FM Systems for People with Impaired Hearing*. New York: New York League for the Hard of Hearing.

Carmen, Richard. 1977. *Our Endangered Hearing*. Emmaus, PA: Rodale Press.

*———. 1983. *Positive Solutions to Hearing Loss*. Englewood Cliffs, NJ: Prentice-Hall. (Chapter 5, ''Lip Reading and Speech Reading,'' is an excellent short course for home study)

Castle, Diane L. 1988. *Telephone Strategies: A Technical and Practical Guide for Hard-of-Hearing People*. Bethesda, MD: Self Help for Hard of Hearing People, Inc.

Clickner, Patricia. ''A Consumer's Guide for Purchasing a Hearing Aid.'' *SHHH Journal*. (May/June 1988):6–8.

Combs, Alec. 1986. *Hearing Loss Help*. Santa Maria, CA: Alpenglow Press.

Dickey, Marilyn. ''How Loud Is It?'' *Washingtonian* (July 1988).

Frankel, George W. 1952. *Let's Hear It*. Hollywood, CA: Stratford House.

Helleberg, Marilyn M. 1979. *Your Hearing Loss*. Chicago: Nelson-Hall.

Howard, Jane. 1984. *Margaret Mead: A Life*. New York: Simon and Schuster.

*Journal of Speech and Hearing Disorders. (Write the American Speech Language Hearing Association at the address given in appendix 4).

*Kaplan, Harriet, Scott J. Bally, and Carol Garretson. 1987. *Speechreading: A Way to Improve Understanding*. Washington, DC: Gallaudet University Press. (All three authors are members of the Gallaudet University faculty)

*Marcus, Irving. 1985. *Your Eyes Hear for You: A Self-Help Course in Speechreading*. Bethesda, MD: Self Help for Hard of Hearing People, Inc.

Mueller, H. Gustav, and Virginia C. Geoffrey, eds. 1987. *Communication Disorders in Aging*. Washington, DC: Gallaudet University Press. (A very technical book, most useful to professionals)

Newby, Hays A., and Gerald A. Popelka. 1985. *Audiology*. Englewood Cliffs, NJ: Prentice-Hall. (An indispensable resource)

Office of Consumer Communications, Food and Drug Administration. 1981. *Tuning in on Hearing Aids*. Rockville, MD: FDA. (Free)

Pulec, Jack L. 1984. "Menière's Disease." In Jerry L. Northern, ed., *Hearing Disorder*, 2nd ed. Boston: Little, Brown.

Rosenthal, Richard. 1975. *The Hearing Loss Handbook*. New York: St. Martin's Press.

Schwartz, Dan. "Hearing Aid Care." *SHHH Journal* (May/June 1988): 9–10.

Simko, Carole Bugosh. 1986. *Wired for Sound*. Washington, DC: Gallaudet University Press. (An excellent primer for hearing-impaired people)

Singer, Jay M., and W. W. Brownell. "Assessment of Hearing Health Knowledge." *Gerontologist* (April 1984): 160–166.

Solomon, Maynard. 1979. *Beethoven*. New York: Schirmer Books.

Superintendent of Documents, U.S. Government Printing Office. n.d. *Hearing Aids*. National Bureau of Standards Monograph 117. Washington, DC: USGPO. (Order no. SN 003-00751-0, §55)

———. 1978. *Facts about Hearing and Hearing Aids*. Washington, DC: USGPO. (Order no. SN 003-02024-9)

Thomas, Alan J. 1984. *Acquired Hearing Loss*. Orlando FL: Academic Press.

U.S. Office of Technology Assessment. n.d. *Hearing Impairment and Elderly People*. Washington, DC: USGPO.

Whitehurst, Mary Wood. 1986. *Listen to Me: Auditory Exercises for Adults*. Washington, DC: Alexander Graham Bell Association for the Deaf.

3447